PHARMACOLOGY

An open learning introduction for healthcare workers

John Sneddon
edited by
Nan Stalker

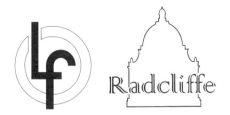

THE OPEN LEARNING FOUNDATION
RADCLIFFE MEDICAL PRESS

USING THIS WORKBOOK

The workbook is divided into 'sessions', covering specific subjects.

In the introduction to each learning pack there is a learner profile to help you assess your current knowledge of the subjects covered in each session.

Each session has clear learning objectives. They indicate what you will be able to achieve or learn by completing that session.

Each session has a summary to remind you of the key points of the subjects covered.

Each session contains text, diagrams and learning activities that relate to the stated objectives.

It is important to complete each activity, making your own notes and writing in answers in the space provided. remember this is your own workbook—you are allowed to write on it.

Now try an example activity.

ACTIVITY

This activity shows you what happens when cells work without oxygen. This really is a physical activity, so please only try it if you are fully fit.

First, raise one arm straight up in the air above your head, and let the other hand rest by your side. Clench both fists tightly, and then open out your fingers wide. Repeat this at the rate of once or twice a second. Try to keep clenching both fists at the same rate. Keep going for about five minutes, and record what you observe.

Stop and rest for a minute. Then try again, with the opposite arm raised this time. Again, record your observations.

▼

Suggested timings are given for each activity. These are only a guide. You may like to note how long it took you to complete this activity, as it may help in planning the time needed for working through the sessions.

▼

Time taken on activity

▼

Time management is important. While we recognise that people learn at different speeds, this pack is designed to take 15 study hours (your tutor will also advise you). You should allocate time during each week for study.

▼

Take some time now to identify likely periods that you can set aside for study during the week.

	Mon	Tues	Wed	Thurs	Fri	Sat	Sun
am							
pm							
eve							

▼

At the end of the learning pack, there is a learning review to help you assess whether you have achieved the learning objectives.

ACKNOWLEDGEMENTS

Writer: John Sneddon, edited (1999) by Nan Stalker

Editor: Tim Burton

Reviewer: Gill Young

Director of Programmes: Leslie Mapp

Programmes Manager: Caroline Pelletier

Production Manager: Stephen Moulds, DSM Partnership

The views expressed are those of the team members and to not necessarily reflect those of The Open Learning Foundation.

The publishers have made all reasonable efforts to contact the holders of copyright material included in this publication.

Radcliffe Medical Press Ltd
18 Marcham Road, Abingdon, Oxon OX14 1AA

British Library Cataloguing in Publication Data

A catalogue record for this book is available from the British Library

ISBN 1 85775 431 X

Typset by DSM Partnership, SW18
Printed and bound by TJ International Ltd, Padstow, Cornwall

CONTENTS

INTRODUCTION

Session One is an introductory session that deals with pharmacology and nursing practice. We introduce the language of pharmacology by looking at the meaning of some of the terms in pharmacology, how drugs are supplied to the public and the law as it relates to nurses and nurse prescribing. The idea of a drug being formulated into a medicine and some of the reasons why this is necessary are explained. The session emphasises the importance of the absorption, distribution, metabolism and elimination of drugs from the body in determining the response to drugs, and takes a look at some of the factors that influence the way in which the patient responds to medicine.

Session Two deals with the principles of the administration of drugs. We look at the different routes used and the advantages and disadvantages for each. The session also introduces the importance of non-pharmacological factors in the response to a medicine. Finally, the idea of drug interactions is introduced.

In Session Three we deal with the factors that influence how the drug moves round the body, from its site of administration until it is finally eliminated.

Session Four introduces the concept of chemical messengers and cell receptors for these messengers. You will learn how important our knowledge of receptors is in the development of new drugs and the targeting of drugs for specific diseases.

Learning Profile

Below is a list of learning statements for this unit. You can use it as a way of identifying your current knowledge and deciding how the unit can develop your learning. It is for your general guidance only. You will need to check each individual session in more detail to identify specific areas on which you need to focus.

For each of the outcomes listed below, tick the box on the scale which most closely corresponds to your starting point. This will give you a profile of learning in the areas covered in each session of this unit. The profile is repeated again at the end of this unit as a learning review, and you will be able to check the progress you have made by repeating it again then.

	Not at all	Partly	Quite well	Very well

Session One

I can:

	Not at all	Partly	Quite well	Very well
• define the meaning of some of the terms used in pharmacology	❏	❏	❏	❏
• explain the application of pharmacology to nursing	❏	❏	❏	❏
• describe the difference between a prescription only drug, a pharmacy medicine and a general sales list medicine	❏	❏	❏	❏
• specify some of the relevant legislation relating to the prescribing of medicines	❏	❏	❏	❏
• explain the professional guidelines relating to nurses and the prescription of drugs	❏	❏	❏	❏
• explain why drugs are formulated into medicines	❏	❏	❏	❏
• explain the importance of the study of pharmacokinetics	❏	❏	❏	❏
• understand the importance of accurate recording and reporting procedures.	❏	❏	❏	❏

Session Two

I can:

	Not at all	Partly	Quite well	Very well
• explain the importance of the different routes of administration of drugs	❏	❏	❏	❏

	Not at all	Partly	Quite well	Very well

Session Two *continued*

- list briefly the advantages and disadvantages of different routes of administration of drugs ❏ ❏ ❏ ❏

- describe the factors that influence the absorption of drugs ❏ ❏ ❏ ❏

- explain the importance of non-pharmacological factors in the response to medication ❏ ❏ ❏ ❏

- show how factors such as weight, gender, age and genetics can influence the response to medication ❏ ❏ ❏ ❏

- explain how some common drug interactions can influence the patient's response to medication. ❏ ❏ ❏ ❏

Session Three

I can:

- explain the key factors influencing the absorption of drugs ❏ ❏ ❏ ❏

- explain how drugs are distributed and eliminated ❏ ❏ ❏ ❏

- describe how drugs are transferred across biological membranes ❏ ❏ ❏ ❏

- explain the role of ionisation in drug transfer ❏ ❏ ❏ ❏

- describe how drugs are transported in the blood ❏ ❏ ❏ ❏

- outline the principles of drug metabolism. ❏ ❏ ❏ ❏

Session Four

I can:

- explain how cells make use of chemical messengers ❏ ❏ ❏ ❏

- explain the concept of drug receptors ❏ ❏ ❏ ❏

- describe the way in which receptors are classified. ❏ ❏ ❏ ❏

The application of pharmacology to nursing

Introduction

In this session we explore the importance of a knowledge of pharmacology to nursing practice. We consider some important legislation and look at the guidelines laid down by the statutory nursing body (UKCC) in relation to professional practice. The basic language of pharmacology is introduced and the terms 'pharmacodynamics' and 'pharmacokinetics' are explored. We discuss the desirable properties of drugs used in human treatment, the formulation of drugs as medicines and the importance of accurate recording and reporting procedures.

Session objectives

When you have completed this session you should be able to:

● define the meaning of some of the terms used in pharmacology

● explain the application of pharmacology to nursing

● describe the difference between a prescription drug, a pharmacy-only medicine and general sales list medicine

● specify some of the relevant legislation relating to the prescribing of medicines

● explain the professional guidelines relating to nurses and the prescription of drugs.

● explain why drugs are formulated into medicines

● explain the importance of the study of pharmacokinetics

● understand the importance of accurate recording and reporting procedures.

1: The importance of pharmacology

This introductory session is called *The application of pharmacology to nursing.* Why do you think nursing students should be required to know any pharmacology? Note down your ideas below.

Commentary

In the past, nurses' responsibility for medication was limited. their responsibility was to ensure that the correct patient received the correct dose by the correct route at the correct time. This ensured that the patient received the medicine as required by prescription. The nurse was not expected to know anything about the nature of the drug or its effect upon the patient.

Today, the nurse is a pivotal member of the healthcare team with increasing responsibility and is expected to exercise judgement in the management of the patient's drug therapy. To do this effectively requires an understanding of drug action and the ability to detect and evaluate both beneficial and adverse responses to drugs.

In the past twenty years, with the development of more potent and selective drugs treatment, protocols have developed that require continual adjustments of the dose and timing of administration to obtain the optimum response for the individual patient. Working within the guidelines of the treatment protocol, this is often done by nurses. We are also seeing the first steps towards 'nurse prescribing'.

In order to carry out these new roles in drug therapy, the nurse must understand drugs. The greater your knowledge of how drugs act, and how they are used in clinical practice, the more you will be able to anticipate drug responses in your patients. This will make you more effective in counselling your patients on their drug therapy, and in optimising their drug administration for maximum benefit.

2: Legislation and professional guidelines

The availability of drugs is strictly controlled by law. The enactment of these laws is the result of a complex interplay of factors. These include:

- issues arising out of drug purity and safety

- factors relating to the monopoly positions of certain professions

- severe laws restricting the possession of certain drugs because they are considered to carry particular risks or because their use is not tolerated socially.

There is no law that requires a drug to be effective in the treatment of the disease for which it is prescribed. However, it is the professional duty of the nurse to be familiar with the laws and regulations relating to drugs and medicines and their administration, and to ensure that their provisions are carried out.

The major laws are the Medicines Act 1968 for prescription drugs and The Medicinal Products: Prescriptions by Nurses, etc. Act 1992 for nurse prescribing. The three ways drugs are made available to patients under the Medicines Act, 1968 are as:

- prescription drugs

- pharmacy only medicines

- over-the-counter drugs.

Prescription only medicines (POMs) are sold or supplied only in accordance with a prescription given by an appropriate practitioner. The practitioner is often a registered doctor but may also be a dentist or a nurse prescriber who may write prescriptions for drugs from a limited list of medicines known as a formulary.

Pharmacy medicines may be sold to the public without a prescription by a pharmacist from registered premises.

General sales list medicines are drugs which may be sold from outlets other than pharmacies.

In addition to these laws, regulations are formulated locally by health authorities or individual trusts and all health districts have their own procedures.

UKCC standards

The United Kingdom Central Council (UKCC) takes the view that registered nurses are competent to administer drugs on their own and to take responsibility for their actions. Nurses' actions in relationship to drug administration are legally covered by their employing authority, when rules and protocols are followed.

The UKCC guidelines state that the nurse must *'carefully consider the dosage, method of administration route and timing of administration in the context of the patient at the operative time'* (UKCC, 1992). This guideline refers to the **pharmacokinetics** of the drug; that is, the processes of drug absorption, distribution and final elimination from the body.

The UKCC requires that all nurses involved in the administration of medicines should:

- have an understanding of substances used for therapeutic purposes

- be able to justify any actions taken

- be prepared to be accountable for the actions taken.

For the nurse, these responsibilities require that his or her knowledge of drug action must be based on a firm foundation of anatomy, physiology, biochemistry and patho-physiology. For example, in order to understand the absorption of a drug after oral administration it is necessary to have knowledge of the anatomy and physiology of the gastro-intestinal tract, the biochemical process of digestion and the factors that influence the passage of small molecules across the cell membranes of the different cells that form the gut wall.

Prescription only medicine: *drugs sold or supplied only in accordance with a prescription given by an appropriate practitioner.*

Pharmacy medicines: *drugs sold to the public without a prescription by a pharmacist from registered premises.*

General sales list medicines: *drugs which may be sold from outlets other than pharmacies.*

Pharmacokinetics: *the effect that drugs have on the human body.*

The objective of drug therapy is to provide the maximum benefit with minimum harm. Nurses have a critical responsibility in achieving this therapeutic objective. In order to meet this responsibility, nurses must understand the pharmacology of drugs.

3: The language of pharmacology

Drug: *a chemical that affects living tissue.*

A **drug** is defined as any chemical that can affect living processes. By this definition, virtually all chemicals are considered drugs, since, when given in large enough amounts, all chemicals will have some effect on living cells. In this unit the term 'drug' is used for those chemicals that have therapeutic applications.

Goodman and Gilman, (1990) define pharmacology thus.

> *'Pharmacology embraces the knowledge of the history, source, physical and chemical properties, compounding, biochemical and physiological effects, mechanisms of action, absorption, distribution, biotransformation and excretion, and therapeutic and other uses of drugs.*
>
> (Goodman and Gilman, 1990)

Given this definition, the science of pharmacology covers a large body of knowledge.

Clinical pharmacology: *the study of the action of drugs in humans.*

Clinical pharmacology is the study of the action of drugs in humans. This discipline includes the study of drugs in patients as well as in healthy volunteers which occurs during new drug development. **Therapeutics** is defined as the medical use of drugs.

Therapeutics: *the medical use of drugs.*

4: Desirable properties of drugs used to treat human illness

New drugs are continually being developed, as most of those presently in use have one or more of the following drawbacks that limit their effectiveness in safely treating human illness:

- they lack potency
- they lack specificity
- they exhibit side-effects.

When developing a new drug, we want that drug to be as good as possible and not attended by any of these drawbacks: in effect, we want the 'perfect drug'. It must be emphasised that such an ideal drug exists in theory only. There can probably never be such a thing as the perfect drug. We need to use our knowledge of pharmacology to make the safest and best use of the drugs currently available and to give informed judgements about the claims made for new drugs.

Three properties are desirable in any drug used to treat a human illness:

- effectiveness
- safety
- specificity.

Effectiveness

Effectiveness (or efficacy) is the essential property of a drug. If a drug is not effective – that is, if it doesn't do anything useful – there is little justification for giving it to a patient.

The clinical effectiveness of many drugs, particularly those used to treat mental illness, where non-drug factors play an important part in the patient's response, is not easy to prove. Much time and money is spent on clinical trails aimed at demonstrating that the administration of a particular drug improves the clinical outcome for the patient.

Safety

There is no such thing as a safe drug. All drugs have the potential to cause injury. What we call a safe drug, then, is one that will not produce harmful effects, even when administered in high doses and for a long time.

The safety of a drug has to be assessed in the light of the seriousness of the condition it is used to treat. The administration of certain classes of drugs is always associated with a known increased risk of side-effects. For example, some anti-cancer drugs that suppress the immune system are associated with an increased risk of serious infection. The balance of the risks is a matter of clinical judgement in the case of each patient. The chances of producing adverse effects to the patient can be reduced by proper drug selection and correct administration, based on a consideration of the pharmacology of the drug.

Selectivity

A selective drug is said to produce only the responses required to treat the disease for which it is given. A selective drug would not ideally produce side-effects. Again, it is important to appreciate that there is no such thing as a selective drug and that all medications have the potential to produce side-effects. Many will do so as the dose administered to the patient is increased.

Additional properties

In addition to the three properties listed above, any drug that is going to be used to treat human illness should, ideally, possess six more that are known to increase the safety margin of drugs.

1   **The action of the drug should be reversible**. Their effects last for a limited time.

2   **The action of drugs must be predictable**. We need to know, with a reasonable degree of certainty, how the patient will respond prior to drug administration. Unfortunately, since each patient has a unique genetic make-up, the accuracy of our predictions cannot be guaranteed. It is one of the responsibilities of the nurse giving medications to monitor the patient's response to drugs. This is particularly important following the administration of a new drug.

3   **The drug should be easy to administer**. This property is important if patients are going to administer the drug themselves. For this reason the preferred route of administration is by mouth. Some drugs, such as insulin, cannot be administered in this way and have to be injected.

4   **The drug should not produce undesirable interaction with other drugs or with constituents of the diet**. Such interactions may either increase or decrease drug responses. For example, diazepam (Valium), a tranquilliser, produces minimal depression of respiration at therapeutic doses. However, if the patient drinks even moderate amounts of alcohol while on the drug, severe respiratory depression may occur. Similarly, the antibacterial effects of the antibiotic tetracycline can be reduced in patients receiving an iron or calcium supplement.

5   **The drug should be cheap to produce**. This ensures that the drug is freely available to all patients who require it.

6   **The drug should be chemically stable**. Some drugs lose effectiveness during storage. Others, which may be stable in powdered form, rapidly lose effectiveness when put into solution. Apart from the cost and inconvenience of discarding and replacing unstable drugs, chemical instability may also give rise to breakdown products that may be toxic or interfere with the therapeutic response to the drug.

5: The formulation of drugs as medicines

Medicine:
a mixture of one or more drugs, combined or formulated with excipients.

Excipients: *inactive constituent of a pharmaceutical preparation.*

It is not normal to administer a pure drug to a patient. Almost all drugs are administered in the form of a medicine. A **medicine** is a mixture of one or more drugs, combined or formulated with other inactive materials known as **excipients**. Excipients themselves have no pharmacological activity but do have a major influence on how the drug is administered and absorbed. The formulation of a drug into a medicine – whether it be in tablet, ointment, injection form or some kind of liquid solution – is usually essential before it can be administered to humans. Each medicine is a highly sophisticated product carefully designed to fulfil its purpose, to ensure that the response to the medicine is the same each time it is administered.

ACTIVITY 2   **// ALLOW 15 MINUTES**

Write down three or four reasons why drugs are formulated into medicines. You may find it helpful to think of the size, shape, colour and form (liquid, injection, tablet, for example) of any medicines that you have seen or administered recently.

Commentary

Your suggestions could have included:

- to increase the stability of the drug so that it is not chemically or biologically altered during storage

- to ensure that each dose contains the correct amount of the drug

- to control the rate of disintegration of a tablet in the stomach, so allowing the drug to be released at the proper rate and in the proper place (usually the small intestine)

- to make the administration of the medicine easier: formulation can be used to disguise a bitter taste or to buffer a drug so that it does not cause tissue damage following injection.

The colour and shape of tablets and capsules are controlled as an aid to identification. Charts are available which allow us to identify all drugs sold as proprietary preparations. The colour of tablets and capsules is also used by manufacturers as a psychological means of increasing the drug's effect. If you look at one of the many drug identification charts available in your hospital pharmacy you will notice that the capsules that contain tranquillisers are in subdued, quiet colours (such as dark greens, blues and even blacks), while the capsules for antidepressants have vibrant colours (such as yellows and reds). These colour combinations are a subtle attempt to enhance the therapeutic effects of the medicine and constitute an example of using the 'placebo' effect in drug administration.

6: Pharmacodynamics and pharmacokinetics

Pharmacodynamics is the term used to describe the effect that a drug has on the body. It determines whether the drug is going to be effective in the treatment of disease with the minimum of side-effects. The initial step leading to a drug response is the binding of a drug to its receptor. This drug receptor interaction is followed by a sequence of intracellular events that results in the response of the cell to the drug.

Pharmacodynamics: *the effect that drugs have on the human body.*

Pharmacokinetics is the term is used to describe the effect the body, its organs and tissues has on the action of a drug once it is administered. It is unusual for the same amount of drug to be eventually available at its site of action. As soon as the drug enters the body, the body will act on the drug to change its concentration and in many cases its chemical structure. In order to be able to use drugs wisely and at the appropriate doses we need to understand the pharmacokinetics of the drug.

Pharmacokinetics: *the process of drug absorption, distribution and final elimination from the body.*

The four major processes by which the body alters the action of a drug are by:

- influencing drug absorption

- influencing drug distribution

- metabolising the drug

- influencing drug excretion.

We will look at these factors later in the unit.

To exert an effect on the body, a drug must reach its target tissue in a suitable form, and in sufficient concentration, to initiate a specific therapeutic effect. Once the pharmacokinetics of a drug are known it is then possible to determine:

- the doses (concentrations) to be given to the patient

- the most effective route of administration

- how frequently the dose has to be given in order to obtain maximum therapeutic benefit for the patient.

The unique characteristics of each patient can influence both the pharmacokinetics and pharmacodynamics processes involved in the drug action. They can also determine the patient's response. Sources of individual variation include:

- interactions between drugs if the patient is receiving more than one drug at the same time

- physiological variables such as age, sex and weight

- patho-physiological variables related to disease (especially reduced function of the kidney and liver, which are the major organs of drug elimination)

- genetic variables which can alter the metabolism of drugs and predispose the patient to unique side-effects which cannot be predicted.

When we consider all of the possible uncontrolled variables associated with the treatment of an individual patient – such as the patient's disease and the multiple pharmacological effects of many drugs – it is easy to believe that any attempt at rational drug therapy is impossible. To the inexperienced and untrained student initial encounters with drug treatment may appear as the best guess on the part of the clinical team backed up by years of clinical experience of what drugs have worked in the past on patients with a similar illness. Fortunately, this is not true. Of all branches of practical medicine it is perhaps the therapeutic aspect of patient care with drugs which is most amenable to objective research. For example we can:

- intervene in the patient's disease with a drug

- objectively measure the response to the drug

- use the data obtained from one group of patients to develop and inform good practice for the use of the drug in other patients.

When we administer a medicine to a patient the active drug itself is only one variable in a complex pattern of events that will determine how that individual patient responds. It is important, therefore, that we spend time considering all of the factors that may happen to our therapeutic objective between the writing of the prescription and the patient's final response to the drug.

ACTIVITY 3 // ALLOW 20 MINUTES

Make a list of as many things as possible that may happen from the writing of the prescription to the patient taking the medicine and the drug being absorbed into the body. Write down everything you can think of no matter how silly it may seem. (I once heard of a patient who would not take their medicine on the thirteenth day of a month because it was unlucky!)

Commentary

I expect that you have written down quite a long list. It is almost impossible for us to work out all of the variables that may influence an individual patient. However, it is important to realise that errors in the administration of medicines are quite common, even by experienced staff.

In clinical practice there are two common sources of error which influence the amount of the drug that the patient actually receives. The first are the medication errors. These usually consist of:

- administering the wrong drug to the patient

- giving the wrong dose or giving the correct dose but at the wrong time.

The second source of error is non-compliance. The patients' ability or desire to continue taking the medicine is one of the most important sources of variability in their response to drug therapy. Common sources of patient non-compliance are:

- patients forgetting to take their medication on a regular basis, so reducing the effectiveness of the treatment

- patients increasing the dose in the expectation that they will get better quicker.

Nurses have a major responsibility in the education of patients on the proper use of their medication. Some of these responsibilities are listed in *Table 1*.

Before administration

Discuss treatment with patient. Explain to the patient what to expect. This is an essential feature of patient education and many patient information leaflets are available to reinforce information given verbally.

Ensure that the prescription refers to that patient.

Apply your knowledge of pharmacology and therapeutics to consider:

- if it is an appropriate drug to give for the patient's condition

- that the prescribed dose and route of administration are appropriate

- the possibility of contra-indications, side-effects and of drug interactions that may occur with any other medication that the patient may be taking.

After administration

Record details of the administration.

Evaluate and assess the patient's therapeutic response.

Record any side-effects.

Continue to support the patient.

Table 1: Responsibilities of the nurse administering medication.
(adapted from White, 1994).

Many aids are available to help patients to maintain compliance. These range from the marketing of tablets and capsules in day-labelled packs to drug holders/dispensers that can be filled by the nurse or the patient and which come marked with both time and day.

ACTIVITY 4   **// ALLOW 10 MINUTES**

Drug dispensers are available from pharmacists and drug suppliers.

- Try to obtain as many examples as you can. The hospital pharmacist may be able to help you with your collection.

- Make a list of the drug dispensers you have found and beside each write down how good it is in assisting the patient with drug compliance.

Remember that many of the patients who require these dispensers are elderly and may have difficulty in seeing or in fine control of their hands and fingers.

Summary

1 In this session you have begun to consider the relationship between pharmacology and nurse practice.

2 You have reviewed some of the legislation and professional guidelines that affect the prescribing of medicines.

3 You have looked at some of the terms used in pharmacology and what they mean. You have found out why drugs need to be formulated into medicines and learnt about the difference between prescription only, pharmacy and general sales list medicines.

4 You have begun to consider the importance of the study of pharmacokinetics.

5 You have considered the importance of accurate recording and reporting procedures.

Before you move on Session Two, check that you have achieved the objectives given at the beginning of this session and, if not, review the appropriate sections.

The administration, absorption, distribution and elimination of drugs

Introduction

In this session we explain the importance of the different routes by which drugs are administered, focusing on administration by mouth, via the mucous membranes, by injection, and by application to the surface of the skin. We also look at the main physiological influences on the way in which drugs are absorbed, and at the effect that drugs can have on one another – focusing particularly on the interaction between drugs and enzymes. We consider factors that are extraneous to the drug, such as body weight, gender and individual response.

Session objectives

When you have completed this session you should be able to:

- list the different routes by which drugs are administered

- explain the advantages and disadvantages of different routes of administration

- describe the main physiological factors that influence patients' responses to drugs

- explain why it is vital to monitor the condition of patients taking more than one drug.

1: Routes for administering drugs

Drugs must be absorbed into the body and transported by the blood to reach their target tissue before they can be effective. The speed at which drugs are absorbed and distributed strongly influences their potency and toxicity.

ACTIVITY 5 // **ALLOW 10 MINUTES**

There is a surprisingly large number of ways in which we can give a drug so that it is absorbed into the bloodstream. Before we look at them, make your own list of possible routes for administering drugs.

Commentary

Almost every possible route of getting drugs into the body is used. The common ones are:

- by mouth – oral administration
- intravenous
- subcutaneous
- intramuscular.

Less common routes include:

- injecting drugs directly into arteries or into a body cavity such as the abdomen
- absorption from under the tongue (sub-lingual administration)
- inhalation through the lungs
- absorption through the mucosa of the rectum or the vagina.

Very specialised routes may include injection into the spinal cord, or application to external organs such as eyes or ears.

Topical administration through the skin can take place when drugs are formulated as lotions or creams.

New methods of drug delivery through the skin include trans-dermal patches and electrophoresis where a weak electric current is used to 'drive' the drug through the skin.

We will now look at each of the common routes in detail.

Administering drugs by mouth

Swallowing is the most common route of drug delivery.

Write down some of the major advantages and disadvantages of oral delivery. Aim to note three or four points in each category.

Commentary

Oral administration is the safest, most convenient and most economical method of drug delivery. Here is a list of the major advantages.

1 The medicine is administered in convenient forms containing the correct dose, for example, in the form of tablets, capsules, or a liquid.

2 Administration does not require sterile preparation or sterile technique.

3 It is the safest method of drug delivery. The drugs can be formulated so they are absorbed at a constant rate from the intestine, reducing side-effects that might occur if the drug was absorbed too quickly.

4 Overdoses are dealt with before absorption is complete, by removing the drug from the stomach.

Here is a list of the major disadvantages.

1 The rate of absorption of the drug from the intestine may be variable and influenced by factors such as the amount of food in the stomach and intestine.

2 The compliance of the patient taking the drug is generally poor. This can be a major problem when the patient is self-medicating. Elderly patients may be confused and forget to take their drugs, or psychotic patients may refuse to take their medication through delusions of poisoning.

3 Many drugs cause irritation to the mucosa of the gastro-intestinal tract. For example, aspirin causes gastric bleeding. The incidence of this type of side-effect may be reduced by using a different formulation of the drug or by taking the drug with food.

4 Many drugs absorbed from the intestine are partially metabolised in the liver before reaching their site of action (the so-called **first-pass effect**). This reduces the amount of active drug reaching its site of action.

First-pass effect: *partial metabolism of a drug by the liver before it reaches the site of action.*

Delivering drugs via external mucosal membranes

Rectal administration

The rectum is a convenient route for administering drugs that would otherwise cause vomiting or excessive irritation to the stomach. Drugs are usually administered in the form of a solid suppository. However, absorption can be irregular and the drug may be expelled from the body with the faeces before it is all absorbed. In addition, the blood from the rectum is not returned to the liver before it enters the general circulation, so about 50 per cent of the drug absorbed from the rectum escapes first-pass metabolism by the liver.

Sub-lingual

The mucosa under the tongue have a very rich blood supply. Since this supply does not pass through the liver before entering the general circulation there is no first-pass metabolism of drugs absorbed from under the tongue. The most common drug administered sub-lingually is glyceryl trinitrate, used for relieving pain in angina (ischaemic heart disease). This is a powerful drug exerting an immediate effect on the heart. However, there is a low risk of overdosing and of side-effects because the drug is completely metabolised in one passage through the liver. This also means that no active drug reaches the heart if the tablet is swallowed accidentally.

Other mucus membranes

Drugs can be absorbed into the body after being applied to other external mucus membranes, such as the nose, ear or vagina. However, these routes are used mainly to deal with local infections or inflammations affecting the organ itself, rather than for general drug administration.

Delivering drugs through the lungs

For drugs (and toxins like tobacco smoke) that are in the form of gases or vapours, inhalation provides rapid and easy access to the circulation due to the large surface area of the pulmonary mucosa. This is obviously important with anaesthetic gases, when there is almost instantaneous absorption of the drug and no first-pass metabolism by the liver. Drug administration direct to the lung is important in local lung disease, such as asthma. The disadvantages of this route are the difficulties in controlling the dose, which could result in overdosing. Also, many volatile chemicals (and drugs) irritate the pulmonary mucosa, causing coughing and inflammation of the lung tissue.

Delivering drugs by injection

Administering drugs by injection is referred to as 'parenteral administration'. Injection into a vein delivers the drug directly into the bloodstream. Drugs are normally injected when other routes of administration are inappropriate and when rapid absorption is required.

ACTIVITY 7 // **ALLOW 10 MINUTES**

List the four most common routes used for injecting drugs.

What do you think will be the effect of the different injection routes on the rate of absorption of the drug?

Commentary

Nurses are normally responsible for administering drugs by the subcutaneous, intradermal or intramuscular routes, and increasingly for the intravenous administration of drugs by injection or infusion.

Intravenous administration

This route delivers a known concentration of drug to its site of action almost immediately. Drugs may be administered rapidly (bolus injection) or slowly over a few minutes. Intravenous administration is also used for delivering fluids and/or drugs that are administered slowly to maintain a constant blood concentration.

Intramuscular administration

This is the deepest of the surface injection sites. Most drugs are easily absorbed following intramuscular injections due to the rich blood supply to muscles and relatively large volumes of drugs can also be injected (1–5 ml).

It is important to choose sites which will not damage major nerves or permit inadvertent injection into a blood vessel. This can be tested by slightly withdrawing the plunger of the syringe before injection to ensure that there is no back-flow of blood – which would occur if the needle had entered a blood vessel. Injections are usually made into large muscle masses such as the upper thigh or the upper part of the buttocks.

Any pain associated with intramuscular injection may be reduced by simultaneously injecting a local anaesthetic. However, this can increase the total volume that has to be injected and may inhibit absorption of the drug by causing vasoconstriction in surrounding blood vessels.

Intramuscular injections may be used for **depot therapy**. This is when a drug is formulated in such a way that it is slowly released over several days or months. Common uses for depot therapy are in administering contraceptive drugs, and anti-psychotic drugs which the patient may refuse to take by mouth.

Subcutaneous injection

This is the injection of drugs into the deepest layers of the skin. Absorption from this site is fast with aqueous solutions of drugs and slower with sustained release preparations. The disadvantage of the route is that it is not suitable for injecting large volumes.

Intradermal administration

This is injection under the skin. It is used mainly for the local administration of drugs. Only small volumes can be injected and absorption into the body is generally poor.

Topical administration

Topical administration involves applying drugs to the surface of external membranes, including the skin. Drugs are normally only applied to the mucosal membranes of the vagina, bladder, eye, nose and other external areas for their local effects on these tissues and not as a method of getting drugs into the bloodstream.

However, drugs can also be applied to the skin as a general method of delivery into the bloodstream. In order to penetrate the many layers of specialised cells that make up the epidermis, drugs have to be soluble in oils or formulated into oily creams or ointments. The oils penetrate the outer layers of the skin and carry the drug into the inner layers where it can enter the blood capillaries. If the skin is damaged or inflamed, then drug absorption is much more rapid due to the breakdown of the outer layers of cells.

Whole body toxic effects are common if highly fat-soluble chemicals come into contact with the skin. This is seen in farm workers who come into contact with lipid soluble insecticides and herbicides formulated in organic solvents. Nerve gases are a group of chemicals designed with a chemical structure that leads to very rapid penetration through the skin.

Recent innovations have extended the use of skin as an administration route. These include the development of controlled-release patches, and electrophoresis – where the local drug is 'driven' through the skin by a mild electrical current.

2: Key physiological factors that influence drug response

As we will discuss later, the body's response to a drug is related to its concentration at its site of action. It is obviously very difficult, if not impossible, to measure the concentration of a drug at its site of action in every patient. Therefore it is normal to estimate the dose required for the 'average' and use this in treatment. This is usually fairly straightforward because the dose-range over which most drugs exert their effects without toxicity is quite large. However, for very potent drugs you may need to refine each dose and relate it to a number of different physiological factors.

Body weight

ACTIVITY 8 // **ALLOW 10 MINUTES**

What influence do you think body weight and body composition may have on a patient's response to a fixed dose of a drug? Make notes of your ideas below before continuing.

Commentary

In a heavy person the 'usual' dose of the drug becomes distributed throughout a larger body mass, which may reduce the concentration of drug at its site of action. This may make it necessary to increase the amount of drug given to a heavy person in order to obtain a satisfactory response. The composition of the body is also important, as fat people can store drugs in their body fat, reducing the therapeutic concentration of the drug at its site of action.

ACTIVITY 9 // **ALLOW 15 MINUTES**

General anaesthetics are lipid soluble drugs (they have to penetrate into the central nervous system). Suppose a general anaesthetic is to be administered to an obese individual for quite a complicated operation. What effect do you think the patient's body composition will have:

● on the time taken for the patient to be anaesthetised

● on the time the patient will have an anaesthetic 'hangover'?

Commentary

As anaesthetics are distributed into the body fat it will take more anaesthetic to induce a fat patient than a thin one. This is because in an obese individual anaesthetic will accumulate in the body fat, and therefore less will be available to penetrate into the brain.

The recovery of the patient will depend to a large extent on the elimination of the anaesthetic. In the obese patient the drug will have to be eliminated from the body fat as well as the brain. This will give rise to a slower recovery time and the residual anaesthetic present in the body fat will delay recovery, giving rise to the anaesthetic 'hangover'.

Age

ACTIVITY 10 // **ALLOW 10 MINUTES**

In what ways do you think extremes of age may influence a patient's response to medicines?

Note down your ideas before continuing.

Commentary

In babies and in very young children the dose of drugs administered has to be monitored carefully as their low body weight means that only low doses of drugs are needed to produce an effect. Babies and young children have a much lower concentration of plasma proteins. These proteins reduce the toxicity of many drugs by binding them so that their active concentration in the plasma is reduced. In addition, the drug-metabolising enzymes in the liver are not fully developed, so more of the active drug is present in the body.

As a result of these factors, babies and young children may show inappropriate responses and toxic effects due to drug overdose unless drug blood levels are monitored carefully.

We encounter other problems of drug administration as we get older. For example, there is an age-related decline in organ function in the liver and kidney. This can lead to altered drug metabolism, distribution and elimination. Overdose effects of the 'standard' dose may be further emphasised by the loss in body mass seen in most elderly people. Bear in mind, too, that many elderly patients tend to be taking a range of drugs and this alone leads to greater drug intolerance and a larger number of toxic interactions.

Gender

ACTIVITY 11 // **ALLOW 10 MINUTES**

Males and females have clear genetic and hormonal differences, as well as generally differing in physical characteristics such as body weight and tissue distribution.

Try to suggest two or perhaps three ways in which you think gender needs to be taken into account when administering a drug.

Commentary

Gender is particularly important in relation to sex hormones used as drugs – for example in hormone replacement therapy.

However, gender can have more subtle effects on individual responses. For example, young males are more prone to sedation from barbiturates than young females. This is due to a lower level of drug-metabolising enzymes in the liver.

These gender differences result from the different effects that androgens (male) and oestrogen (female) have on different drug-metabolising systems in the body. In females the activity of the enzymes in the liver, which metabolise a wide range of drugs, can be stimulated by oestrogen. However, women appear to be more susceptible to adverse drug reactions than men. Chloramphenicol-induced aplastic anaemia is twice as common in women than in men, and phenylbutazone-induced agranulocytosis three times as common in women than in men.

Gender differences in the response to drugs are rare before puberty and disappear after the menopause.

An additional example is reproduced in *Resource 1* which details the exploration into the effect on mortality of the use of combined oral contraceptives.

Genetic differences

ACTIVITY 12 // **ALLOW 10 MINUTES**

We all differ physiologically as a result of our genetic makeup. This makeup also influences the way in which our bodies handle drugs. See if you can note down how this influence might occur.

Commentary

The drug-metabolising enzymes in the liver are under the control of more than one gene. The patterns of their hereditary influence are complex and can be quite widespread in a population.

At least ten families of genes are known in humans for the important drug-oxidising enzymes known as the cytochrome P450 system. One result of this is that the rate at which a drug is oxidised (metabolised) in the liver can vary significantly between individuals and between races. In Caucasians approximately 90 per cent of the population have the genetic makeup that allows them to extensively and rapidly metabolise a wide range of drugs. However, 10 per cent of this population are poor metabolisers. These individuals experience severe side-effects to the drug even at normal therapeutic doses, as they are not able to metabolise and eliminate the drug in the time recommended between successive doses.

A dramatic example of the effect of enzyme induction on drug response is seen in barbiturates. These drugs can induce sedation in humans, and in overdose produce respiratory depression and death. Before the ability of these drugs to produce drug dependence was fully appreciated they were widely used as sleeping pills. Patients who took them regularly became rapidly tolerant to the sedative effects and had to keep increasing the dose. In some patients this meant they could tolerate several hundred times the normal lethal dose.

Illness

ACTIVITY 13 // **ALLOW 10 MINUTES**

Organ or tissue damage resulting from illness may alter the distribution and elimination of a drug or have an effect on the patient's sensitivity to it. Many patients with severe or prolonged illness experience impaired functioning of their liver and kidney.

How do you think this will affect the body's response to drugs? Write down your ideas below.

Commentary

The majority of drugs are metabolised in the liver to inactive metabolites so any impairment of liver function may lead to reduced drug metabolism. This causes the active drug to accumulate in the body, resulting in a more prolonged and intense action. There is also an increase in side-effects as the drug builds up in the tissues. Impairment in the function of the kidney would have a similar effect, as the drug would not be excreted in the urine. This would also lead to the drug accumulating in the body, prolonging its action and increasing the incidence of side-effects.

3: The effect of drug interactions on patient response

In many chronic illnesses it is normal to treat the patient with more than one drug at a time. This approach is often essential, because in severely ill patients there is usually more than one disease or group of symptoms, each of which may need treating simultaneously with different drugs.

Many drug combinations that are prescribed to treat such patients are based on sound pharmacological principles. For example, in patients with cardiac failure it is often essential to stimulate the heart with a drug such as digoxin and at the same time give the patient a diuretic drug to stimulate urine flow, preventing the build up of oedema.

In cancer chemotherapy, and in treating most infections, multiple-drug therapy with different drug combinations prevents the emergence of malignant cells or bacteria that are resistant to the effects of the drugs.

Although there is nothing inherently wrong in giving a patient a combination of drugs, you should be aware that drug combinations greatly increase the probability of side-effects – sometimes with fatal consequences. For this reason, you need to keep the rationale for giving a patient more than one drug under continuous review.

A number of drug-drug interactions are well known. It is the responsibility of the nurse administering medicines to be aware of them so that they do not adversely affect the patient. Charts and cards are available which list these common adverse drug interactions, and these charts should be displayed in all wards or clinics where drugs are dispensed.

The incidence of adverse drug interactions in patients with multiple drug therapy is not known. Estimates of the proportion of hospitalised patients showing some side-effects range from two per cent to 30 per cent. In the community the estimates range from nine per cent to 70 per cent of all patients. It has been estimated that in 20 per cent of all patients receiving ten or more drugs the side-effects are so severe that the symptoms of the side-effects are being treated by one of the drugs being given to the patient. The average hospitalised patient is probably receiving eight to ten drugs, so the problem of drug or therapy induced disease could be large. The nurse responsible for treating the patient needs to be aware of this and to discuss any new or untoward symptoms that appear with the medical staff and the pharmacists.

Enzyme induction as an example of drug–drug interactions

Earlier in this session we mentioned the enzyme system cytochrome P450. Can you remember where it is mostly found in the body and how its levels are controlled?

Write down anything you can recall and then check your notes against the commentary below.

Commentary

Cytochrome P450 is an important drug-metabolising enzyme system present in the liver and in other organs where drug metabolism takes place such as the intestine and the kidney. The amount of this enzyme system in the body is under the control of multiple genes.

The amount of enzyme in the body can also be increased by exposure to any of a wide range of chemicals in a process termed **enzyme induction**. When this occurs the rate of metabolism of all drugs oxidised by this enzyme is increased, decreasing the duration of the drug's action and resulting in therapeutic failure.

Enzyme induction: *an increase in enzymic activity resulting from exposure to any of a wide range of chemical agents.*

Drugs which are powerful inducers of drug-metabolising enzymes in the liver are:

● the barbiturates

● the anticonvulsant drugs, such as phenytoin and carbamazepine.

Drugs whose action can be reduced by enzyme induction include:

● oral anticoagulants. The reduced effect of anticoagulant activity leads to increased incidence of pulmonary embolism.

● low-dose oestrogen contraceptives. An increased rate of metabolism leads to lower tissue concentrations and contraceptive failure.

● theophylline. Accelerated metabolism leads to decreased blood concentrations and increased asthmatic symptoms.

Enzyme inhibition as an example of drug interactions

As we have already noted, side-effects can occur when a drug increases enzyme activity. Toxic interactions can also occur when a drug inhibits essential enzyme systems in the body. Some drugs are specifically designed to inhibit enzymes.

Bacteria and other micro-organisms have different metabolic pathways from humans. Advantage is taken of this fact to design drugs that affect essential enzymes in bacteria but have no effect on humans. A number of anti-virus drugs and anti-cancer drugs also act as enzyme inhibitors.

One example of an enzyme-inhibiting interaction occurs when administering the anti-depressant drugs known as monoamine oxidase inhibitors (MAOIs) which are used as anti-depressants. Monoamine oxidase is an important enzyme which is present in every cell except red blood cells. The highest concentrations of the enzyme occur in the gut, liver and kidney. Its main function is to metabolise a large number of molecules known as amines which are either present in our food, particularly in cheeses and nuts, or produced as the result of the digestion of proteins.

If these amines enter the bloodstream they produce a dramatic and dangerous rise in blood pressure. Our protection against this is the monoamine oxidase present in the cells of the intestine and liver which metabolise the amines before they can reach the general circulation.

ACTIVITY 15	// ALLOW 10 MINUTES

What advice would you give a depressed patient just starting a course of treatment with an MAOI?

Commentary

The MAOI will inhibit monoamine oxidase throughout the body. This removes the protection given by the monoamine oxidase in the cells of the intestine and liver against tyrosine and other amines produced by digestion. After eating amine-containing foods, large mounts of amines could enter the bloodstream resulting in a dangerous rise in blood pressure.

It is essential to explain to patients on these drugs why they must not eat certain foods while they are on medication, and to provide them with a list of these foods. The list includes cheeses, red wine, marmite and other meat extracts, beans and many cooked and prepared meats. These foods are high in tyrosine and other amines which can raise blood pressure.

In addition to the interaction with some foods, MAOIs interfere with the metabolism of a number of drugs and increase their effects. These include pethidine, the barbiturates, amphetamines and some anaesthetics.

Because of the potential fatal effects of these interactions with MAOIs, patients must be drug-free for at least three weeks before any new or changed drug therapy is introduced.

The interaction of MAOIs and diet is sometimes known as the cheese effect. It was first reported by a pharmacist who was prescribed a new drug (one of the first MAOIs) for the treatment of depression. He was also partial to a cheese sandwich and a glass of milk before he went to bed. He found that after starting on his new medication he woke up about an hour or so after eating his cheese sandwich with a severe headache and racing pulse. He did not experience these symptoms if he stopped his medication or gave up his cheese sandwich at night. Subsequent laboratory research worked out the mechanism of the toxic interactions between MAOIs and tyrosine produced from the diet.

ACTIVITY 16 // ALLOW 20 MINUTES

Next time you are on a ward, compare the patients' drug charts with one of the published lists or charts of known adverse drug combinations.

If you do notice such a combination, discuss it with the medical staff or the clinical pharmacist. Do not jump to the conclusion that someone has been careless in prescribing. There are often good clinical reasons why 'unsuitable' combinations are prescribed for individual patients.

Binding to plasma proteins

There is another important aspect of drug interaction that may influence response. A large number of drugs are transported in the blood bound to plasma proteins. During the time it is bound to plasma proteins the drug is not in 'free' solution and cannot diffuse out of the blood to reach its site of action. As a result, the drug has no pharmacological action or therapeutic effect. Plasma proteins are therefore an important storage site for drugs, slowly releasing them as they are required. However, the number of available binding sites on the plasma proteins is limited. If these sites are already occupied by one drug and the patient is administered another drug that binds to the same site, then the new drug may compete with and displace the first drug.

ACTIVITY 16 // ALLOW 10 MINUTES

Imagine that a patient has been stabilised on a fixed dose of a drug which is quite toxic. Fortunately, the drug is strongly bound to plasma proteins from which it is slowly released to exert its therapeutic effect, so with normal doses the blood levels are never high enough to be toxic. Suddenly, the patient's condition changes and it is decided to add another drug to the treatment. This new drug unfortunately combines with the original treatment for plasma binding sites.

What would be the consequences for the patient? Write down your ideas below.

Commentary

A potential drug interaction occurs when a patient receives two drugs which bind to the same site on the plasma proteins. In this case, the introduction of a new drug will displace the original drug from its binding site, leading to a sudden and dangerous rise in the free concentration of the drug in the blood and tissue fluids. This is the equivalent of giving a massive overdose, resulting in extra effect and duration of action with the possibility of an increased incidence of side-effects.

A well-documented example of this type of interaction occurs with the anticoagulant drug Warfarin. This drug is mostly bound to plasma proteins but it is easily displaced from its binding sites by a number of other drugs, including aspirin. The result is potentially dangerous blood levels of Warfarin, leading to a greatly increased risk of severe internal bleeding.

Summary

In this session you have considered the importance of the different routes by which drugs are administered, and looked at some of the main advantages and disadvantages of different routes.

You have learned about the main physiological influences on the way in which drugs are absorbed, and the effect that drugs can have on one another.

Before you move on Session Three, check that you have achieved the objectives given at the beginning of this session and, if not, review the appropriate sections.

SESSION THREE

Pharmacokinetics and drug action

Introduction

In this session we will consider some of the factors clinical pharmacologists take into account when deciding the most appropriate dose and frequency of administration of a new drug. We begin by building on your work in previous sessions on the physiological aspects of drug action, and then look in more detail at the transport of drugs around the body, with particular emphasis on the process of ionisation and the role of enzymes.

Session objectives

When you have completed this session you should be able to:

- explain how the body absorbs, distributes, metabolises and eliminates drugs

- describe how drugs are transferred across biological membranes

- explain how the chemical properties of drugs influence their absorption

- explain the role of ionisation on the movement of drugs

- use a simple formula to measure the distribution of a drug in the body.

1: Pharmacokinetics

Clinical pharmacokinetics is the study of the absorption, distribution, metabolism and elimination of drugs over time, and how these processes are related to the duration of the pharmacological response. Knowledge of the pharmacokinetics of a drug is essential in order to work out:

● when to expect the maximum response to a drug after administration

● how long a drug will stay in the body

● how frequently to administer a drug in order to maintain a therapeutic response.

In all countries that have strict legislation controlling the safety and purity of drugs, it is impossible for a manufacturer to put a new drug on the market without providing evidence that the metabolism, distribution and excretion of the drug and its major **metabolites** (breakdown products) are understood. This information is essential to allow us to make rational choices about the dose of drug, how frequently it should be administered and at what concentrations we are likely to see toxic effects.

Metabolites: the breakdown products of a drug.

Before a new drug is administered to patients a great deal of information will be available on its activity and toxicity. This information will come from:

● animal studies

● phase I studies on a small number of individuals (usually 50–200).

The purpose of a phase I study is not to find out whether a drug is active, but to administer low doses and study its metabolism and elimination. This information is used to calculate the doses to be used in clinical trials in patients. It is at this stage that the new drug is evaluated for its clinical effects and some estimate made about the incidence and severity of any side-effects.

Pharmacokinetic information is not available for all the drugs that we use. This is particularly true for the 'older drugs'. Also, the information available for an individual drug represents an 'average' value for all the humans on which the drug was tested. Because those tested tend to be healthy, young (usually male) individuals (phase I clinical trials) it may be necessary to individualise the dose. It takes time to build up experience in how best to use a new drug in a more mixed patient population.

Pharmacokinetics should help us to predict side-effects that are related to the dose of the drug. This is why the nurse's role in patient observation is important, especially if the patient is being administered a new drug for the first time.

The administration 'experiment'

If you are responsible for administering medicines it is important to take the time to understand the principles behind the absorption, distribution and elimination of the drugs and how their concentration in the body relates to their action. This is part of the broad base of pharmacological knowledge that will help you to make the appropriate judgements and achieve a therapeutic outcome. However, you should always be aware that drug administration is a step into the unknown.

ACTIVITY 18 // **ALLOW 15 MINUTES**

You are working in a medical unit and a clinical pharmacologist is about to start treating a patient with a new drug. In the briefing beforehand the pharmacologist says to the team: 'Every time you administer a drug to a patient it is an experiment.' List two or three reasons why he or she might say this.

Commentary

The clinical pharmacologist will have a good idea of the dose to be administered and how the drug is metabolised and excreted. He or she may even know what to expect in the way of adverse reactions. However, the factors that make drug administration an 'experiment' include:

● the fact that each patient comes with his or her own genetic makeup

● the nature of the patient's illness.

As a result, the first administration of a drug to a patient requires more care and attention than a repeat dose after the patient has been receiving a drug for some time.

2: Factors influencing drug bioavailability

The availability of a drug at its site of action is influenced by a number of factors. Two of the most important are:

● the drug's rate of metabolism and excretion

● the rate at which the drug is absorbed from its site of administration.

The bioavailability of a drug is influenced primarily by the way the drug is metabolised by the liver. Drugs that are absorbed from the stomach or intestine must pass through the liver before they reach the general circulation. The liver is the major organ of drug metabolism, where the majority of drugs are metabolised to inactive metabolites. Therefore, even if the drug is 100 per cent absorbed from the intestine, some will be metabolised in the liver before it can reach its site of action. You will recall that this decrease in bioavailability is called 'the first-pass effect'.

When pharmacologists talk about the absorption of a drug into the body they are describing:

- the rate at which a drug leaves its site of administration (i.e. oral or injection)

- the extent to which this occurs.

For most routes of administration it is unsafe to assume that 100 per cent of a drug will be absorbed after administration. This can be particularly true after oral administration or the application of a drug to the skin in the form of a cream or ointment.

From the point of view of treating the patient, the amount of drug actually absorbed is not all that important providing we know:

- how much is absorbed after a particular method of administration

- that there is no large variation between the responses of individual patients.

What is important is the amount of drug that actually reaches its site of action in the body.

Factors influencing absorption

ACTIVITY 20 // **ALLOW 15 MINUTES**

List two or three key factors which you think may influence the absorption of drugs. Focus on administration, which we have already discussed, but try to extend your list to cover factors specific to a drug or its formulation.

Commentary

Absorption of drugs is influenced by many factors. These include:

- **concentration**. Drugs administered in high doses or concentrations tend to be absorbed faster.

- **the area of the body surface available**. The lung has a large surface area available for the absorption of drugs, so drugs administered in the form of gases or vapours are absorbed through the lung into the bloodstream at rates equivalent to an intravenous injection. Part of the attraction of 'crack cocaine' is that it can be administered rapidly through the lung to produce the same 'rush' as an intravenous injection but without the same dangers of infection.

- **the clinical state of the patient**. A patient who is in shock will have reduced blood flow to the skin and muscles. This will slow the absorption of drugs from superficial injection sites.

You may also have suggested the following factors related to the properties of individual drugs:

- solubility

- specific chemical properties.

We will now look at these factors in a little more detail.

Drug properties and drug absorption

Absorption depends partly on the solubility of the drug. Medicines that are already dissolved in solution are more rapidly absorbed than those given in the form of suspensions or capsules. So the formulation of the medicine can have an important influence on drug absorption.

The chemical properties of the drug are also important. Drugs that are acids, such as aspirin, are poorly absorbed from the stomach because they are poorly soluble in the acid gastric juice. Many drugs are designed to be slightly acid so that they will be absorbed from the upper section of the small intestine and not the stomach.

ACTIVITY 20	// ALLOW 10 MINUTES

Imagine a clinical situation where a patient is in shock. Suggest two possible routes by which you can quickly administer drugs.

Commentary

Quick routes include intravenous injection or inhalation (in the latter case the drug would need to be formulated into a nebulised spray). Drug absorption from injection sites in the skin or muscles sites is increased by improving local blood flow by massage or applying heat to the site of injection.

3: Drug distribution

After a drug has been administered, sufficient must be available at its site of action and at an appropriate concentration to produce a therapeutic effect. This depends on the dose administered and on the ease with which the drug can move round the body. Here we focus on the second of these two factors.

The passage of drugs through cell membranes

The body is made up of a number of tissues and organs, each composed of a large number of different cells. When drugs move between different organs and tissues they need to pass through these different cell membranes.

ACTIVITY 21　　　　　　　　　　　　　　**// ALLOW 25 MINUTES**

Plot (in the form of notes or a flowchart) the journey of a drug through the body after oral administration until the drug and its metabolites are eliminated in the urine. Show the major organs that the drug will enter and leave on its journey.

Commentary

The drug will first dissolve in the fluids of the intestine. To be absorbed into the blood it has to pass across the membranes of the cells lining the wall of the gut and then the cells that form the blood capillaries. On reaching the liver it passes back across the wall of the blood capillaries, leaving the blood to enter the liver cells. Here some of the drug is metabolised to water soluble metabolites.

To leave the liver the drug and/or its metabolites have to cross the cell membrane of the liver cells and enter the blood again. When the drug reaches the kidney it passes across the capillary cell membrane and enters the cells of the kidney. The metabolites (and some drug) pass out of the kidney cells into the urine. For the majority of drugs and their metabolites the kidney is the major excretory organ. This is why administering drugs to patients with renal disease is monitored carefully to avoid a toxic build-up in the body due to impaired excretion.

The movement of a drug through cell membranes is influenced by the chemical and physical properties of its molecules. The most important of these properties are:

● size and shape. The smaller the size of the molecule the easier it will be for the drug to diffuse across cell membranes.

● solubility of the drug at its site of absorption.

Some drugs use specialised transport processes to enter cells. However, the majority of drugs cross cell membranes by simple diffusion. As the cell membrane is composed mostly of two layers of specialised fats or lipids, known as phospholipids, the ease with which the drug diffuses across a cell membrane is related to its solubility in oils.

ACTIVITY 22	// ALLOW 10 MINUTES

General anaesthetics are lipid soluble. Suggest why this property is important for the effect of this class of drugs on the cells in the brain.

Commentary

For a general anaesthetic to get into the brain it has to diffuse across a large number of cell membranes, first from the lung into the bloodstream (most general anaesthetics are gases); then from the bloodstream into the brain. The greatest barrier to diffusion into the nerve cells will be the fatty myelin sheath that surrounds the neurones. To penetrate through the myelin sheath the drugs have to be lipid soluble.

Chemistry revision

The next part of this session looks some of the key chemical properties of drugs that influence their action on the body. If you are unsure about the way in which molecules form ions and the properties of ions, then you should work your way through the chemistry revision section, (*Resource 2* in the *Resources Section*) before continuing with this session. If you feel confident about these concepts, continue with the text .

The effect of ionisation on the diffusion of drugs across cell membranes

When dissolved in water or body fluids, many drugs dissociate into ions and behave either as weak acids or bases. Assume that drug A is slightly acid when in solution (such as aspirin). It will dissolve in water and give a mixture of the non-ionised drug HA and a positively-charged cation H^+ (which is the hydrogen ion), and the drug A^- which has a negative charge. When this occurs we say that the drug is ionised.

$$HA \rightleftharpoons A^- + H^+$$

The double arrows indicate that an equilibrium, or balance, exists between the two forms. When dissolved in water, drug A will exist mostly in the ionised form A^- and H^+ with only a small number of the non-ionised molecules HA present.

As the non-ionised forms of drug molecules are lipid soluble, drug A is poorly absorbed from those areas of the intestine where it exists mostly in its ionised form.

ACTIVITY 23	// ALLOW 15 MINUTES

The relationship between the amount of ionised and non-ionised drug in solution is the key to our understanding of drug movement through the body. Using the information concerning the ionisation of aspirin, write down why you think that a drug which is fully ionised may be poorly absorbed.

Commentary

Most drugs ionise in solution and behave as weak acids or bases. As only the non-ionised form of a drug is lipid soluble, it is this form of the drug that most easily penetrates cell membranes.

We can use this information to look now at the effect of ionisation on the absorption of drugs from the intestine.

How ionisation influences absorption from the gastro-intestinal tract

The stomach is a hostile environment for most chemicals. Its acid secretions mean that its contents have a pH of about 1.5. This low pH not only affects the stability of some drugs, but also has a major influence on their ionisation. This can be used to advantage: it is possible to ensure that drugs are not absorbed in the stomach, but are absorbed further down the intestine where the conditions for efficient absorption are better.

After swallowing, our drug A will pass into the stomach and dissolve in the gastric juice. In the stomach the hydrochloric acid is almost completely ionised to give the two ions H^+ and Cl^-.

$$HCl \rightleftharpoons H^+ + Cl^-$$

In solution our drug A would also ionise.

$$HA \rightleftharpoons H^+ + A^-$$

When ionised, both the hydrochloric acid and drug A would produce the hydrogen ion, H^+. However, in the stomach there is already a high concentration of H^+ from the hydrochloric acid. This makes it difficult for drug A to ionise, which means that in the acid stomach a greater proportion of drug A remains in the non-ionised form, HA.

ACTIVITY 24 // ALLOW 5 MINUTES

If most of the drug in the stomach is in the non-ionised form, what effect will this have on its absorption?

Commentary

As the non-ionised form of the drug HA is the lipid soluble form of drug A, it can now diffuse across the cells of the stomach and enter the bloodstream. In this way, the stomach is able to absorb drugs that are slightly acid and soluble in gastric juice. (You have already noted that many acid drugs are poorly absorbed from the stomach because they are not very soluble in gastric juice.)

Drugs that dissolve in water to give a slightly alkaline solution are not absorbed from the stomach. The explanation for this is as follows.

Our second drug is known as 'B' (for 'basic', or alkaline in solution). It will dissolve to give a slight alkaline.

$$BOH \qquad B^+ + OH^-$$

non-ionised   ionised

Note: an excess of H^+ in solution makes that solution acid (pH less than 7); an excess of OH^- (hydroxyl ions) makes the solution alkaline (pH greater than 7).

When our drug B is swallowed, a small amount dissolves in the acid contents of the stomach.

$$HCl \qquad H^+ + Cl^-$$

$$BOH \qquad B^+ + OH^-$$

In the presence of the hydrochloric acid the ionisation of drug B is increased.

ACTIVITY 25 // ALLOW 10 MINUTES

Can you suggest why the ionisation of the drug BOH is increased in the stomach? Note down your response below.

Commentary

The reason is that the H+ ion from the hydrochloric acid and the OH– ion from the drug BOH combine to form water (H_2O). This leaves the ionised form of the drug, B+, in the gastric juice. In this form the drug cannot diffuse across the cell membranes of the stomach wall so it is not absorbed from the stomach.

When the drug passes from the stomach into the intestine, the opposite sequence of ionisation takes place. The fluid in the intestine is alkaline, at about pH 8, with an excess of OH– ions. Some of these will combine with the ionised form of the drug, B+, passing from the stomach into the intestine.

$$B+ + OH– \ BOH$$

As the form BOH is non-ionised it is now lipid soluble enough to cross the cell membranes of the intestine into the bloodstream and be absorbed from the intestine.

ACTIVITY 26   // **ALLOW 20 MINUTES**

We have just seen why only the non-ionised form of a drug in solution can diffuse across a cell membrane. This may be difficult to understand the first time round. Take a piece of paper and work back though the example you were given for drug BOH. Work out for yourself the influence of the pH from the stomach and from the small intestine on the absorption of the drug.

Commentary

The first step is to recall that the diffusion or penetration of a drug through cell membranes is related to the lipid solubility and the degree of ionisation of the drug when it is in solution. It is the non-ionised forms of the drugs which are lipid soluble and which can penetrate or diffuse across cell membranes.

When drugs dissolve in water they form negatively-charged and positively-charged ions.

$$AH \rightleftharpoons A^- + H^+$$

for a drug that behaves as a weak acid in solution.

$$BOH \rightleftharpoons B^+ + OH^-$$

for a drug that behaves as a weak base in solution.

Drug absorption from the stomach proceeds as follows.

There is an excess of H^+ due to the ionisation of hydrochloric acid in the gastric juice.

$$HCl \rightleftharpoons H^+ + Cl^-$$

This high concentration of H^+ from the acid prevents the ionisation of drugs that are slightly acid by suppressing the formation of the positively charged ions by the drug.

$$AH \rightleftharpoons A^- + H^+$$

Thus, in the stomach most of the drug AH will exist in the non-ionised form. As this form of the drug can diffuse across the cell membranes of the stomach wall into the bloodstream, drugs that ionise like this will be absorbed from the stomach.

Drug absorption from the intestine is influenced by the fact that the digestive juices are alkaline so that they contain an excess of OH^-. This suppresses the ionisation of drugs that behave as weak bases in solution.

$$BOH \rightleftharpoons B^+ + OH^-$$

Thus, in the intestine most of the drug BOH exists in its non-ionised form. This is the form which can diffuse across the cell membranes of the intestine wall into the bloodstream.

How drugs are transported in the blood

If drugs were transported in simple solution in the water of the blood plasma, they would be excreted rapidly by the kidney and their action would be of short duration. Instead, most drugs are bound loosely, and in a reversible manner, to binding sites on the plasma proteins. The drug bound to plasma protein is in equilibrium with the unbound or 'free' drug in the plasma water, so this binding acts as a reservoir from which the drug is released over time. Only the small proportion of the drug that is free in solution can diffuse throughout the body water to reach its site of action.

$$\text{Drug bound to plasma proteins} \rightleftharpoons \text{Drug 'free' in plasma water}$$

The binding of drugs to plasma proteins is one of the body's major influences in determining:

● how long drugs remain active

● their side-effects.

In order to understand the importance of this binding of drugs it is important to appreciate that when a drug is bound to the plasma protein it cannot diffuse to its site of action, and therefore has no pharmacological activity. Only the unbound 'free' fraction of the drug has any pharmacological activity or is capable of being metabolised and eliminated from the body.

There are two important features of plasma binding to remember.

1   If a drug is 99 per cent bound to plasma proteins then only one per cent will be in solution and pharmacologically active.

2   As the one per cent that is free is metabolised and secreted, more of the drug will be released from the plasma protein to maintain the ratio between bound and unbound drug. In this way binding creates a reservoir from which the drug is slowly released.

Plasma binding and drug toxicity

All drugs bind to the same binding sites on the plasma proteins. This can give rise to significant interactions between drugs that bind to the same sites and can lead to toxic interactions. We have already seen that an example of this type of interaction occurs between the anticoagulant drug Warfarin and aspirin. Let's look at the mechanism of this interaction in a little more detail.

Warfarin is a useful drug in preventing vascular clotting in venous thrombosis and pulmonary embolism. It is also a toxic drug (it is used as a rat poison) which in overdose can result in bleeding into the joints and under the skin, leading to marked bruising.

About 99 per cent of Warfarin is bound to plasma proteins. If the free concentration of Warfarin in the blood rises more than a few per cent then there is a serious danger of excessive bleeding. In severe cases, there may be a fatal bleed. For this reason the bleeding time in patients on Warfarin is monitored carefully. Danger is normally avoided by adjusting the dose so that the plasma binding sites are not fully occupied. Then they can act as a 'sink' or reservoir to bind the slight excess of Warfarin that occurs after each administration of the drug.

Warfarin is an acidic drug. If the patient takes any other acid drug while taking Warfarin this drug displaces Warfarin from its binding sites on the plasma proteins. The levels of free Warfarin in the body fluids can then rises to an extent that may lead to a fatal bleed. This interaction occurs when a patient on Warfarin also takes aspirin or oral antidiabetic agents.

A great deal of information is available about the displacement of one drug from plasma protein binding sites by another. Detailed information is available from dispensaries. Staff involved in administering medicines, or advising patients, can obtain charts listing the dangerous combinations from a hospital or regional drug information unit.

4: The principles of drug metabolism

The activity of a drug in the body is normally terminated by metabolism in the liver and elimination of the metabolites in the urine. A major consequence of metabolism is that the drug is converted into more water soluble products that are more easily excreted through the kidney.

The proportion of drug excreted unchanged in the urine varies. Some drugs are not metabolised at all (such as amphetamine). In this case the termination of their activity is determined by the rate of elimination in the urine.

The metabolism of drugs takes place at several sites in the body. Name the most important organ and suggest two or three other organs that may also metabolise drugs.

Commentary

The enzyme systems responsible for the metabolism of most drugs are located in the liver cells (remember the first-pass effect that reduces the bioavailability of drugs absorbed from the intestine). In addition to the liver, drug-metabolising enzymes are present in the gastro-intestinal tract, lung and kidney. These organs also metabolise drugs, although less effectively than the liver. The lung appears to be the main site of metabolism for some circulating hormones such as angiotensin.

Within the tissues drugs, like every other chemical, are subject to alteration (**biotransformation**) by the enzyme systems present in the body. The products of these enzymatic reactions (metabolites) have properties different from the original compound. As a result of these reactions, pharmacological activity can be:

Biotransformation: *alteration of chemical compounds by the enzyme systems of the body.*

- decreased – most metabolites are less active when compared with the original drug

- increased – some drugs are converted in the body to the active compound, or the metabolite is more active than the original drug: such drugs are called **pro-drugs**

Pro-drugs: *conversion of a drug to its active compound by enzymic activity.*

- unchanged – a small number of drugs are not metabolised, but excreted unchanged.

In general, the biotransformation of drugs in the body terminates the action of drugs by producing inactive metabolites. This is not chance; the medicinal chemist 'designs' new drugs to be metabolised and the pharmacological activity of the major metabolites has to be established before a new drug can be licensed for human use. *Table 2* summarises the activity of four major drugs and their metabolites.

Drug	Transformation	Action of metabolite
l-Dopa (inactive pro-drug)	activation (in brain)	dopamine (neurotransmitter)
paracetamol	oxidation (in liver)	toxic metabolites
amphetamine	not metabolised	no change
codeine	metabolised to morphine	more active

Table 2: Some examples of altered drug activity by biotransformation.

The pathways for drug metabolism in the liver

Metabolism in the liver occurs in two phases. Phase I reactions metabolise the drug to a more water-soluble metabolite, mostly by enzyme reaction involving oxidation of the drug. The metabolite formed is usually less active than the parent drug, so Phase I reactions are very important in terminating the activity of drugs.

Phase II reactions are also called conjugation reactions. These reactions link the metabolites of the Phase I reactions with substances such as glucuronic acid that make them water soluble. The conjugated metabolites are easily excreted in the urine.

ACTIVITY 28 // **ALLOW 10 MINUTES**

Note down two major functions of the drug metabolising systems in the liver.

Commentary

One function of drug metabolism is to terminate the activity of the drug. The second function is to produce metabolites that are more water soluble than the parent drug so that they are excreted by the kidney more easily.

The liver did not evolve to metabolise drugs. The major function of the powerful enzymatic activity of the liver is to protect the body from the many toxic substances we ingest with our food, or which are produced during metabolism. Many of the substances absorbed from the intestine enter the portal circulation and have to pass through the liver before entering the general circulation. It is this 'first-pass' metabolism that degrades many chemicals before they reach the general circulation.

5: The elimination of drugs and their metabolites

The body eliminates drugs either unchanged or in the form of its metabolites. Excretion in the urine is most common, but there are other pathways, such as the lungs, faeces and sweat glands. It is important to appreciate that if drugs or their metabolites are eliminated inefficiently the result may be disease or damage to the liver or kidney. This can in turn lead to the rapid accumulation of toxic concentrations.

ACTIVITY 29 // ALLOW 10 MINUTES

Imagine that a friend has come to visit, several hours after eating a meal heavily spiced with garlic. What two pathways are being used to eliminate the volatile components of garlic, and what other major pathways may also be involved?

Commentary

The major organ of elimination for the volatile components is the lung, although a secondary route is excretion onto the skin through the sweat glands. Other metabolites which are water soluble are excreted by the kidney. The garlic and its residues not re-absorbed from the intestine will be eliminated from the body with the faeces.

ACTIVITY 30 // ALLOW 10 MINUTES

Before a drug is licensed for use, it is a requirement that the proportion of the administered dose that is excreted unchanged is known. Why do you think this should be so important? Note down your ideas below.

Commentary

It is important to know how much of the active drug is excreted unchanged because any change in the pattern of excretion due to disease or organ damage will have a profound effect on the therapeutic response to the drug. For example, clinical studies on healthy individuals may indicate that 70 per cent of a drug is excreted unchanged (not metabolised) in the urine. This information can be used to calculate how frequently the drug should be administered to maintain satisfactory blood levels. However, in patients with impaired kidney function, the drug will be excreted at a slower rate and the dosage can be adjusted accordingly. As kidney function generally decreases with age, different doses of a drug that is excreted mostly unchanged may be used in young and old patients.

Factors involved in the elimination of chemicals by the kidney

The majority of drugs and their metabolites dissolved in the plasma water are filtered as the blood passes through the glomerulus of the kidney. Because the drugs and metabolites are in a water soluble form they cannot diffuse back across the kidney membranes into the blood and are eliminated with the urine.

A small number of drugs are actively secreted by the renal tubules into a filtrate that forms the urine. This occurs with the elimination of penicillin and with other drugs such as morphine.

When the plasma is filtered at the kidney glomerulus, most of the water, and nutrients such as glucose present in the filtrate, are re-absorbed back into the bloodstream further along the kidney tubule. In a similar manner, some drugs are re-absorbed into the blood after being removed by filtration. This can prolong the activity of these drugs in the body. Most water soluble drugs are not re-absorbed by the kidney but some lipid soluble drugs, such as the inhalation anaesthetics, are almost completely re-absorbed by the kidney and therefore not excreted by that route.

For a number of drugs and their metabolites the kidney is more than a filter that removes the chemicals from the plasma. The kidney has important functions controlling the blood levels of ions such as sodium and nutrients such as glucose. These physiological mechanisms can also affect the excretion of drugs.

The kidney is an important organ in maintaining the acid-base balance in the body, and this in turn influences the excretion of chemicals. The kidney also adjusts the excretion of H+ and HCO3 in the urine to maintain the pH of the blood within constant limits.

ACTIVITY 31   **// ALLOW 10 MINUTES**

What influence do you think the pH of the urine will have on the re-absorption of drugs that are ionised in the filtrate? It will help you to think about the earlier discussion of the effect of ionisation of a drug on its passage through a cell membrane.

Commentary

The pH of the urine will affect the passive re-absorption of a chemical by influencing the amount of the non-ionised form present in the kidney filtrate. Acid drugs, such as aspirin, are excreted at a faster rate in an alkaline urine. This increases the proportion of the drug in the ionised form which does not easily diffuse from the filtrate into the renal tubule. If the urine were acid, more of the non-ionised form would be present and it is possible that some of the aspirin would be re-absorbed.

ACTIVITY 32	// ALLOW 10 MINUTES

Using the information given in the previous activity, how do you think you could increase the elimination of (a) aspirin (b) amphetamine in the urine of patients admitted with an overdose?

Commentary

(a) As aspirin is an acid drug that is filtered by the kidney in a water soluble form, you could increase excretion by making both the blood plasma and the kidney filtrate slightly alkaline. This would increase the proportion of the drug which was ionised. You could achieve this by giving the patient sodium bicarbonate.

(b) For amphetamine (a basic drug), renal elimination increases if the blood and urine are slightly acid, increasing the ionisation of the amphetamine. You can achieve this by giving the patient a mild acidic salt such as ammonium chloride.

6: Measuring the distribution of drugs in the body

The body is composed of a large number of organs, tissues, cells and fluids. Any one of these – for example the heart or brain – can be referred to morphologically and functionally as a compartment. However in terms of pharmacokinetics the word **compartment** refers collectively to all organs, tissues, cells and fluids in which the uptake and distribution of a drug is identical. For example, if we administered radioactive water it would rapidly equilibrate with all intracellular and extra-cellular water in the body. If we measured its concentration it would appear that the body only consists of one water compartment. This contrasts with the way in which we view body water distribution in an anatomical sense. In this case we distinguish blood from another fluid compartment such as cerebral spinal fluid.

Compartment: *organs, tissues, cells and fluids in which the uptake and distribution of a drug is identical.*

Body water is distributed into several compartments. In the normal, lean male weighing about 70 kg, water comprises about 58 per cent of body weight; that is, about 41 litres. The extra-cellular water is about 12 litres and included within this is about three litres of circulating plasma water. The whole blood volume, including the intracellular water of the erythrocytes, is twice the plasma volume; that is, about six litres.

Clearance: *the rate of removal of a drug from the body.*

The **clearance** of a drug is its rate of removal from the body (usually measured in minutes or hours). In most treatment situations you will want to keep the drug concentrations at a steady state within the blood concentration to produce the best response. If 100 per cent bioavailability is achieved with a drug then such a steady state is reached when the rate of drug elimination is exactly balanced by the rate at which the drug is being administered.

Volume of distribution: *a measure of the distribution of water in which a drug has become distributed within the body.*

The **volume of distribution** (Vd) of a drug is a measure of the volume of water in which the drug has become distributed within the body (compartment). Vd is relatively simple to determine. A known amount of a drug is administered, and after allowing sufficient time for it to distribute, a sample of blood is taken and the concentration of the drug determined.

If the drug was distributed without metabolism, elimination or binding, then the determination of the volume of distribution could be compared to finding the volume of a fluid by adding a known amount of dye and measuring its concentration after thorough mixing.

How to calculate the volume of distribution (Vd)

Example 1

A 50 mg dose of a drug is injected into a 70 kg man and a plasma concentration of 1 mg/litre is calculated at zero time (i.e. when the drug has become uniformly distributed, in practice about three minutes after injection). What is the volume of distribution?

Answer

To give a final concentration of 1 mg/litre the drug must be distributed in 50 litres of body water. Therefore, Vd = 50 / 1 = 50 L or approximately total body water.

Example 2

One g (1000 mg) of a drug is administered by intravenous injection. After a few minutes, to allow the drug to become distributed throughout the body, the concentration in plasma was 0.3 g/ml-1. What is the volume of distribution?

Answer

Vd = 1000 / 0.3 = 3000 ml or 3 litres. This suggests that the drug is distributed in a volume equal to the plasma water.

ACTIVITY 33 // **ALLOW 5 MINUTES**

After injection, the Vd for a drug indicates that it is distributed in a volume of about three litres. Write down below what this tells us about the distribution of the drug in plasma.

Commentary

A volume of distribution of three litres is equivalent to the plasma volume. This tells us that the drug is 'stuck' in the plasma and is not becoming distributed throughout the body. It suggests that the drug is strongly bound to the plasma proteins.

When we study the pharmacokinetics of drugs and their metabolites in patients we usually mean the study of the plasma levels and how they change with time after drug administration. The reason for this is that the blood is easily accessible. Sensitive chemical methods exist to determine the blood levels of most known drugs. The simplest example of a pharmacokinetic study is to administer a known concentration of a drug by rapid intravenous injection and to measure the blood concentration over a series of time points.

Summary

In this session you have learnt how the chemical properties of drugs influence their absorption and subsequent transport round the body.

You have found out about the transfer of drugs across cell membranes, and the effect of ionisation on this process, and looked at how drugs are transported in the blood and eliminated by the body.

Finally, you have considered the principles of drug metabolism, particularly in relation to the liver and kidney, and reviewed some of the practical applications of pharmacokinetics.

Before you move on to Session Four, check that you have achieved the objectives given at the beginning of this session and, if not, review the appropriate sections.

SESSION FOUR

How drugs act

Introduction

In this session we will look at some of the ways the body uses chemical messengers to communicate between different cells and to co-ordinate the activities between individual cells and tissues. We will look both at the release of messages, and at their interpretation by specialist protein molecules called receptors. We will also consider the effect that certain drugs, such as nicotine, can have on these mechanisms.

The processes we will be exploring can go seriously wrong in human disease, and this provides a major target for drug action and the development of effective treatment.

Session objectives

When you have completed this session you should be able to:

● explain how cells communicate with one another

● outline the relevance of receptors to drug action

● describe the way in which receptors are classified.

1: Mechanisms for drug action

Once a drug is administered and absorbed into the body it has to exert a pharmacological action before it is effective in relieving the patient's illness. Most drugs act by one of only three major mechanisms.

1. **They replace or mimic the effects of a natural chemical messenger in the body.** An example of this type of activity would be administering the drug L-Dopa to patients with Parkinson's disease. In the brain the dopa is converted into the neurotransmitter dopamine.

2. **They block or prevent the actions of a chemical messenger.** An example of this is administering adrenergic blocking drugs to block the effect of adrenaline in patients with heart disease. This results in a decrease in the work done by the heart.

3. **They inhibit (and more rarely stimulate) enzymes.** An example of this type of action is the use of monoamine oxidase inhibitors to treat depression.

Cell signalling

The human body is made up of hundreds of thousands of living cells, many of them highly specialised. They are grouped together in tissues and organs. These cells and groups of cells carry out the vital functions that are essential for life. In order for the body to work properly these cells have to communicate with one another to regulate their development, growth and organisation and to co-ordinate their functions in both health and disease.

The concept of communication between cells helps us to understand the mechanisms of many diseases and how we can treat these with drugs. For example, hydrochloric acid secretion in the stomach is controlled by histamine produced by cells in the gastric mucosa. Blocking the action of histamine on acid secretion is a major treatment for gastric ulcers.

Generally, communication between cells uses one of three basic signalling systems:

- gap junctions

- signalling molecules

- chemical secretion.

Gap junctions

Gap junctions:
'holes' in the cell membr anes between two cells through which the cytoplasms of the cells can make contact.

Gap junctions are 'holes' in the cell membranes between the two cells though which the cytoplasm of the cells can make contact. The cells can then communicate by:

- chemical signals in the form of small molecules that diffuse through these gap junctions between the cells

- electrical signals that pass through the gaps.

The muscle cells of the heart are connected by gap junctions. In heart cells these junctions form areas of low electrical resistance so that the electrical impulses generated in the pacemaker regions of the heart can reach all of the heart cells rapidly. This results in synchronising the electrical coupling of the heart cells so that all muscle cells in a particular chamber of the heart contract at the same time. This forces the blood out of the chamber. When heart cells are damaged after a heart attack, this electrical coupling may break down and the chambers of the heart may not beat as a unit. As a result, the patient may suffer heart failure.

Signalling molecules

Cells also have signalling molecules on their surface. These influence the behaviour of the other cells when they are in direct contact. An example of this type of communication is the adhesion molecules that 'glue' cells together to form tissues and organs. In some types of cancer the adhesion molecules do not work properly and the cancer cells can detach themselves from the original tumour. They are carried around in the body until they stick to another organ and may grow into secondary tumours.

Chemical secretion

Cells can communicate by secreting chemicals which transmit a chemical message from one cell to another, sometimes over quite large distances. This is one of the body's most common forms of internal communication. It is used:

- in the endocrine system

- by the nerve cells of the peripheral and central nervous systems

- in the immune system

- for local communication between different types of cells that are close together but not directly touching.

Cell signalling and drug action

Most drugs used to treat human illness achieve their therapeutic effect by interacting with one or more of these three signalling systems. For example, many of the drugs used to treat mental illness, neurological diseases such as epilepsy, and cardiovascular disease, act on the chemical messenger systems in the nervous system.

A great deal of research is now being carried out on newly discovered signalling systems such as the adhesion molecules and similar signalling molecules expressed on the surface of cells. The reason for this is that many of these signalling molecules are thought to be important in the cell signalling associated with the immune system. When they do not work properly they are involved in the development of arthritis, coronary heart disease and transplant rejection.

In the remainder of this session we will be looking in more detail at cell communication using chemical messengers. This is because intervening in the activity of chemical messengers, either by enhancing it, or more usually by blocking it, is a very fruitful way of developing new drugs.

2: Chemical messengers as a method of cell communication

Chemical signalling is a convenient way for cells to communicate. When a suitable cell is stimulated, it responds by releasing a chemical which diffuses through the tissue fluid. In order to detect and recognise these different chemical messengers, cells have evolved specialised protein molecules called receptors in their cell membranes. They usually respond by altering their shape when the messenger binds to active sites on the molecule.

The body uses chemical signalling in three ways:

- synaptic signalling

- endocrine signalling

- paracrine signalling.

Synaptic chemical signalling:
chemical transmission between the cells in the nervous system and between nerve cells and other cells such as muscle cells.

Receptor: *a specialised receiving agent located on the cell surface.*

Synapse: *a specialised gap or junction at nerve endings across which chemical transmission takes.*

Neurotransmitter: *a chemical messenges within the autonomic nervous system.*

Endocrine chemical signalling: *hormone secreting cells secrete their chemical messengers directly into the bloodstream.*

Paracrine chemical signalling: *chemical transmission between paracrine cells which release a local hormone and tissue cells close to the paracrine cell.*

Synaptic chemical signalling is the name given to chemical transmission between the cells in the nervous system and between nerve cells and other cells such as muscle cells. About twenty different chemicals are used as chemical messengers by different nerves, although the process is identical in all nerves.

Stimulation of a nerve releases a chemical from the nerve ending which acts as a chemical messenger. The chemical transmitter diffuses across the small gap between the nerve ending and the next cell to act on specialised **receptors** on the cell surface. When the chemical messenger combines with its receptor it starts a series of events that leads to the cell responding in an appropriate way. The specialised gaps or junctions across which this type of chemical transmission takes place are called **synapses** and the chemical messengers are termed **neurotransmitters**.

In **endocrine chemical signalling**, hormone-secreting cells release their chemical messengers (hormones) directly into the bloodstream. The hormones travel in the blood to act on target cells that may be widely distributed throughout the body.

Paracrine chemical signalling also involves a hormone. In this case, specialised cells called paracrine cells release a 'local' hormone, but this only diffuses a short distance in the tissue to influence tissue cells close to the paracrine cell. These local hormones are not normally found in blood.

3: Revision of chemical transmission in the autonomic nervous system

There now follows a brief revision section on the autonomic nervous system. It is important to understand the basic concepts of chemical transmission between nerves and their effector organs because drugs that alter the normal process of synaptic transmission are those chosen for the treatment of most diseases.

The major physiological functions of the sympathetic and parasympathetic nervous system are given in *Table 3*. This is provided as a convenient summary that you can refer to, if necessary, as you work through the remainder of the unit.

Organ	Sympathetic nervous system	Parasympathetic nervous system
heart	increased rate and force of contraction	decreased rate and force of contraction
smooth muscle of bronchioles	relaxation	contraction
smooth muscle of the pupil	dilation (mydriasis)	contraction (meiosis)

Organ	Sympathetic nervous system	Parasympathetic nervous system
gastro-intestinal tract	decreased peristalsis	increased peristalsis
smooth muscle of the bladder	relaxes; prevents urination	contracts; assists urination
bladder sphincters	contracts; prevents urination	relaxes; permits urination
metabolism	increases levels of glucose	none
blood vessel to the skin and viscera	constrict	none
blood vessels to muscle	dilates	none
adrenal gland	releases the hormone adrenaline	none
sweat glands	thick secretion	watery secretion
salivary glands	thick secretion	watery secretion
hair muscles	contraction	none

Table 3: Functions of the autonomic nervous system.

The parasympathetic nervous system

The chemical transmitter in all sections of the parasympathetic nervous system is acetylcholine. Acetylcholine is located at the synapses in the parasympathetic ganglia and at the synapse at the end of the post-ganglionic parasympathetic nerve fibre. Acetylcholine acts on different types of receptors at these two sites.

In the ganglia, acetylcholine acts on a post-synaptic receptor called the nicotine receptor. It is called the nicotine receptor because the stimulant effects of acetylcholine on the post-ganglionic nerve are mimicked by nicotine. These receptors are blocked by ganglionic blocking drugs.

ACTIVITY 34 // **ALLOW 15 MINUTES**

When we smoke we absorb nicotine that stimulates the autonomic ganglia. List one response that would result from stimulation of the nicotinic receptors in:

● the sympathetic ganglia

● the parasympathetic ganglia.

If you are unsure of the different responses look back at *Table 3*.

Commentary

Nicotine stimulates the nicotinic receptors for acetylcholine and nerve impulses pass down the post-ganglionic nerve fibre to stimulate the end organs. Stimulation of the sympathetic ganglia raises blood pressure. One effect of stimulating parasympathetic ganglia is to increase the flow of saliva. Both of these effects are seen in smokers.

In the synapse at the post-ganglionic nerve ending, acetylcholine stimulates the contraction of smooth muscle or the secretion of glands by acting upon the muscarinic receptors. At this receptor site the actions of acetylcholine are mimicked by the drug muscarine, but not by nicotine. These receptors are blocked by atropine and similar drugs.

ACTIVITY 35	// ALLOW 10 MINUTES

Many drugs block the muscarinic receptors as a side-effect to their main therapeutic use. Usually the side-effects are relatively trivial (in pharmacological terms), but because of discomfort and inconvenience to the patient they are of major concern. Look at *Table 3*. List two or three side-effects that would result from blocking the muscarinic receptors that may cause problems during therapy.

Commentary

Drugs that block the muscarinic receptors produce a dry mouth, urinary retention and blurred vision, all of which greatly inconvenience the patient.

The sympathetic nervous system

The chemical transmitter at the post-ganglionic sympathetic nerve ending is noradrenaline. Stimulation of the sympathetic nervous system not only results in the release of noradrenaline from the post-ganglionic sympathetic nerve endings but also adrenaline from the medulla of the adrenal gland. When the hormone adrenaline is released into the bloodstream it has widespread effects throughout the body. These reinforce the effects of sympathetic nerve stimulation.

Activation of the sympathetic nervous system, and the release of adrenaline, are the major chemical messengers responsible for the increases in heart rate, sweating and the other physiological response that we associate with the stress response.

ACTIVITY 36 // ALLOW 15 MINUTES

The physiological effects of sympathetic stimulation are widespread throughout the body and involve the actions of both adrenaline and noradrenaline. Consult *Table 3* and list the major physiological responses to sympathetic stimulation.

Commentary

You could have summarised the main effects as follows:

- contraction of smooth muscle (blood vessels, pupil of the eye)

- stimulation of both the force of contraction and heart rate

- relaxation of smooth muscle (blood vessels and bronchioles)

- stimulation of the metabolism of stored fat to fatty acids and glycogen to glucose.

These different physiological responses to the same chemical transmitter and hormone are mediated by different receptors.

- Contraction of smooth muscle (i.e. blood vessels, pupil of the eye). These effects are the result of stimulating alpha (a)-receptors located on the smooth muscle cells. The a-receptors are stimulated by the neurotransmitter noradrenaline, and less effectively by the hormone adrenaline.

- Stimulation of both the force of contraction and heart rate. This effect is the result of stimulating a beta (ß)-receptor located on the heart muscle cells. This receptor is stimulated by adrenaline and is termed the ß1-receptor.

- Relaxation of smooth muscle (i.e. blood vessels and bronchioles). This effect is the result of stimulating another type beta (ß)-receptor located on the smooth muscle cells. This receptor is stimulated by adrenaline and is termed the ß2-receptor.

- Stimulation of the metabolism of stored fat to fatty acids. This effect is the result of stimulating a third type of ß-receptor located on fat cells. This receptor is also stimulated by adrenaline and is termed the ß3-receptor.

4: Classifying receptors

Receptors are classified according to the actions of the chemical messenger that stimulates them. One of the major research areas in pharmacology is the classification of the different types of receptors found in the body. The reason for this is that by understanding the response produced by stimulating the different types of receptors we can develop new drugs that are more selective in treating disease and that have fewer side-effects.

The precise classification of receptors is important for, as we have seen with acetylcholine and noradrenaline, there is often more than one type of receptor for each chemical messenger.

Sub-types of receptors

The major types of receptors can be divided into sub-types each of which responds differently to the same chemical messenger.

The classification of these different sub-types of receptors is not just a pharmacological curiosity; it has important implications for drug development. As each receptor sub-type is a different protein, encoded by a different gene, it should be possible to develop drugs that are selective for only one receptor sub-type. For example, adrenaline can act on all three receptor sub-types. It stimulates:

- the ß2 receptor, to relax smooth muscle. Drugs that stimulate this receptor are used to dilate the bronchiole smooth muscle during an asthmatic attack

- the ß1 receptor, which in turn stimulates the heart. Drugs that block this receptor are used in the treatment of angina

- the ß3 receptor, to increase fat metabolism. There are currently no drugs available that selectively stimulate this receptor. However, they are being developed as potential slimming agents.

The symptoms of many diseases result from a wrong or inappropriate response to a chemical messenger acting at one of its receptor sites. An understanding of how these different receptors produce different types of cellular response may enable us to design drugs that interact selectively with these receptors to reverse disease or reduce symptoms.

This approach to the development of new drugs has been successful over the last twenty years. Examples include:

- the development of the histamine H2 blocking drugs in the treatment of gastric and duodenal ulcers

- the ß1 blocking drugs for hypertension and heart disease

- ß2 stimulating drugs in the treatment of asthma

- the development of a new drug, sumatriptan, used in the treatment of migraine. This drug acts by selectively blocking a receptor sub-type (the five HT1 receptors) located on the cerebral blood vessels. This reduces the vasodilatation in the intracranial blood vessels and relieves the headache and other symptoms associated with a migraine attack.

Agonists and antagonists

Some chemical messengers and drugs bind to receptors and activate them to produce a measurable biological response. These are termed **agonists**. Drugs that bind to receptors but do not activate are called **antagonists**. The binding of an antagonist to a receptor occupies the binding sites on the receptor, preventing the chemical messengers or drugs binding to and activating the receptor. Drugs with either agonist or antagonist properties are widely used in medicine. An essential characteristic of the antagonists used in medicine is that their effects must be easily reversible.

The significance of receptor mechanisms

The physiological action of a chemical or drug on a living organism depends on its chemical structure and properties. Fortunately for us the majority of chemicals occurring naturally have little or no effect on the vital activities of our bodies. However, the situation is different with drugs. These are chemicals discovered by chance or designed to affect the activities of living cells, usually by interacting with receptors for chemical messengers or with essential enzymes.

As we have already seen, receptors can exist in a variety of sub-types which are responsible for mediating the different physiological responses produced by the relatively small number of hormones and neurotransmitters found in the human body. With the majority of chemicals used as drugs, the pharmacological activity of the chemical is closely related to its chemical structure. Small changes in structure can have dramatic effects on pharmacological activity. A detailed understanding of receptor sub-types and the physiological responses they produce allows us to develop new drugs or to modify existing ones, so that they are more active and selective, with fewer side-effects. In this way, we can continue to make major therapeutic advances.

Summary

In this final session you have found out how chemical messengers are used as a method of communication between different types of cells in the endocrine system, the paracrine system and the synapses.

You have learnt about the role of drug receptors and how these receptors are classified.

You have considered how drugs that act on receptors can be used to combat certain sorts of disease.

Finally, you have noted how the receptors for chemical messengers occur in families and looked at the different effects exerted by members of the same family.

Agonist: *a drug that binds to receptors and activate them into producing a measurable response.*

Antagonist: *a drug that binds to receptors but does not activate a response.*

LEARNING REVIEW

You can use the list of learning outcomes given below to test the progress you have made in this unit. The list is an exact repeat of the one you completed in the beginning. You should tick the box on the scale that corresponds with the point you have reached now and then compare it with your scores on the learning profile you completed at the beginning of the study. If there are any areas you are still unsure about you might like to review the sessions concerned.

	Not at all	Partly	Quite well	Very well

Session One

I can:

- define the meaning of some of the terms used in pharmacology ❏ ❏ ❏ ❏

- explain the application of pharmacology to nursing ❏ ❏ ❏ ❏

- describe the difference between a prescription only drug, a pharmacy medicine and a general sales list medicine ❏ ❏ ❏ ❏

- specify some of the relevant legislation relating to the prescribing of medicines ❏ ❏ ❏ ❏

- explain the professional guidelines relating to nurses and the prescription of drugs ❏ ❏ ❏ ❏

- explain why drugs are formulated into medicines ❏ ❏ ❏ ❏

- explain the importance of the study of pharmacokinetics ❏ ❏ ❏ ❏

- understand the importance of accurate recording and reporting procedures. ❏ ❏ ❏ ❏

	Not at all	Partly	Quite well	Very well

Session Two

I can:

- explain the importance of the different routes of administration of drugs ❏ ❏ ❏ ❏

- list briefly the advantages and disadvantages of different routes of administration of drugs ❏ ❏ ❏ ❏

- describe the factors that influence the absorption of drugs ❏ ❏ ❏ ❏

- explain the importance of non-pharmacological factors in the response to medication ❏ ❏ ❏ ❏

- show how factors such as weight, gender, age and genetics can influence the response to medication ❏ ❏ ❏ ❏

- explain how some common drug interactions can influence the patient's response to medication. ❏ ❏ ❏ ❏

Session Three

I can:

- explain the key factors influencing the absorption of drugs ❏ ❏ ❏ ❏

- explain how drugs are distributed and eliminated ❏ ❏ ❏ ❏

- describe how drugs are transferred across biological membranes ❏ ❏ ❏ ❏

- explain the role of ionisation in drug transfer ❏ ❏ ❏ ❏

- describe how drugs are transported in the blood ❏ ❏ ❏ ❏

- outline the principles of drug metabolism. ❏ ❏ ❏ ❏

Session Four

I can:

- explain how cells make use of chemical messengers ❏ ❏ ❏ ❏

- explain the concept of drug receptors ❏ ❏ ❏ ❏

- describe the way in which receptors are classified. ❏ ❏ ❏ ❏

RESOURCES SECTION

Contents

Resource 1

The British Journal of Family Planning 1998: 24: 2-6

The effects on mortality of the use of combined oral contraceptives

Katerine Oldfield – *Research Assistant*
Ruairidh Milne – *Visiting Senior Lecturer in Public Health Medicine,*
Wessex Institute for Health Research and Development, University of Southampton, Southampton SO16 7PX, UK
Martin Vessey – *Professor of Public Health*
Department of Public Health and Primary Care, University of Oxford, UK.
(Accepted January 9 1998)

Summary

<u>Objective</u>. To assess, using a computerised mode, the effects on mortality of the use of combined oral contraceptives (COCs).

<u>Design</u>. Two hypothetical cohorts of one million women each, identical except for their use of contraception. The impact of COC use was explored by applying, to each cohort, death rates which were adjusted according to a series of assumptions about the risks associated with COC use. The model also explored the effects of a number of different patterns of COC use.

<u>Settings and subjects</u>. Women aged 16, followed through to ages 50 and 75, exposed to 1994 UK death rates.

<u>Main outcome measures</u>. Numbers of deaths from various cancers and cardiovascular diseases attributable to COC use.

<u>Results</u>. Based on the standard pattern of use, there were 1.7 per cent more deaths in the COC cohort to age 50. The important effects on mortality of different patterns of use and of different assumptions about risks in ex-users were illustrated.

<u>Conclusions</u>. The results confirm the findings of earlier work and provide some reassurance about the likely adverse effects of COC use.

Introduction

In the 1989 Jephcott Lecture at the Royal Society of Medicine, an overview was presented of the benefits and risks to health of use of combined oral contraceptives.[1] The overview attracted considerable interest and, in 1991, a computer model was developed which allowed the analysis to be extended and refined.[2]

The results of this analysis provided reassurance about the likely net effect of COC use on mortality, but highlighted the sensitivity of the model to different assumptions about risk, particularly in relation to breast cancer. For instance, of the three breast cancer risk assumptions, only the worst produced an excess in the total numbers of deaths before age 75.

Since then, new evidence has emerged about the adverse effects of COCs, in two areas in particular. In October 1995, evidence suggesting that use of two of the newer 'third generation progestogens' – gestodene and desogestrel – is associated with an increased risk of venous thromboembolism in comparison with older progestogens was presented to the Committee on Safety of Medicines in the United Kingdom[3] and subsequently published.[4-7] Later, in June 1996, the results of a meta-analysis of world wide epidemiological evidence on the relationship between breast cancer risk and the use of COCs were reported[8]

This report presents the results of a further development of the model, to take account of this new evidence and to explore a further range of assumptions about risk and patterns of COC use.

Methods

The model. The model considered two hypothetical cohorts of one million women each, followed from their 16th to 75th birthday. The groups were assumed to be identical except for their use of contraception. The effects of COC use were examined in relation to death from a number of causes: five cancers (ovarian, breast, cervical, endometrial and liver): four cardiovascular diseases (acute myocardial infarction (AMI), cerebral thrombosis (CT), venous thromboembolism (VT) and subarachnoid haemorrhage (SAH)); and deaths associated with IUD use and sterilisation, as well as maternal mortality.

The model explored the impact of varying assumptions about the relative risk of these conditions associated with COC use. These assumptions were assumed to depend on past duration of exposure and to persist, for variable lengths of time, in ex-users. The effect of varying contraceptive failure rates was also explored.

Death rates and contraceptive failure rates. Death rates for all causes and for COC-related causes were calculated from the national age-specific numbers of deaths and the estimated resident population in England and Wales for 1994.[9] Table 1 shows the ICD-9 codes used.

Disease	ICD-9 code	Description
Cardiovascular diseases		
Acute myocardial infarction	410	
Cerebral thrombosis	433–434	Cerebral infarction
	435	Transient cerebral ischaemia
	436	Acute but ill-defined cerebrovascular disease
Venous thromboembolism	415.1	Pulmonary embolism
	451–453	Phlebitis, thrombophlebitis, venous embolism and thrombosis
Subarachnoid haemorrhage	430	
Cancers		
Breast	174	Malignant neoplasm of female breast
Cervix	180	Malignant neoplasm of cervix uteri
Ovary	183	Malignant neoplasm of ovary and other uterine adnexa
Liver	155	Malignant neoplasm of liver and intrahepatic bile ducts
Endometrium	182.0	Malignant neoplasm of corpus uteri, except isthmus
Maternal		
	630–676	Complications of pregnancy, childbirth and the puerperium
Other		
IUD		Deaths associated with the use of intra-uterine devices
Sterilisation		Deaths associated with sterilisation

Table 1: Causes of death (with ICD-9) code) explored in the model.

Pattern	COC age of use	IUD age of use	Sterilisation at age
A	16 to 24	25 to 34	35
B	**16 to 29**	**30 to 39**	**40**
C	16 to 34		35
D	16 to 39		40
E	16 to 49		

Table 2: Patterns of contraceptive use analysed in the model.

The emboldened row (pattern B) was taken as the 'standard' pattern of use

The maternal death rate was calculated from the age-specific numbers of obstetric-related deaths and numbers of maternities for 1994 (estimated from the number of live births and number of terminations).[9-10]

IUD-related death rates were calculated using North American data which suggest between 1.3 and 2.9 deaths per 100,000 woman years of use.[11] A one-off lifetime risk of four deaths per 100,000 was assumed for sterilisation.[11]

Contraceptive failure rates per thousand woman years were assumed to be five. 10 and 50 for COC, intrauterine devices and condoms respectively. Higher contraceptive failure rates of 10, 20 and 100 respectively were also investigated.

Patterns of contraceptive use. The effects of five patterns of COC use were investigated. These are shown in Table 2. Pattern B (shaded) was taken as the 'standard' pattern of use: that is, COC use from 16 top 29 years, IUD from 30 to 39 years and sterilisation at age 40. The effects of different sets of risk assumptions were analysed using this pattern of use. The effects of the other patterns of use were explored for a standard set of risk assumptions and for the various breast cancer risk assumptions.

Assumptions about disease risk

Cancer. Three assumptions were explored for breast cancer, based on the results of the recently published overview of the association of breast cancer with hormonal contraceptives[8] (Table 3). These included the central results of the overview (B1) together with the lower and upper 95 per cent confidence limits (B2 and B3 respectively). Three assumptions were also explored for cervical cancer, two each for liver and ovarian cancer, and one for cancer of the endometrium. These assumptions included no change in risk; risk changed in current users only; and risk changed in current and ex-users. In addition, three assumptions were explored for cervical cancer; two (C1, C2) were used and explained previously [1,2] and the third (C3) was added as an intermediate position. The two assumptions tested for liver and endometrial cancer were also explained previously. Two assumptions were examined for ovarian cancer, one was used previously (O1); and an alternative assumption, of reduced long-term benefit, was also looked at (O2).

Description of risk	Duration Of use	Relative risk*	After stopping
Liver			
L1 No increased risk			
L2 Risk increases with			
Duration of use	**<=7yrs**	**1.00**	
Risk persists in ex-users	**>=8yrs**	**4.50**	
Breast			
B1 Risk in current users		**1.24**	
Risk persists in ex-users		**1.16**	**1-4yrs**
		1.07	**5-9yrs**
		1.00	**>=10yrs**
B2 Low risk in current users		1.15	
Risk persists in ex-users		1.08	1-4yrs
		1.02	5-9yrs
		1.00	>=10yrs
B3 High risk in current users		1.33	
Risk persists in ex-users		1.23	1-4yrs
		1.13	5-9yrs
		1.00	>=10yrs
Cervix			
C1 No increased risk			
C2 Risk increases with			
duration of use	**<=2yrs**	**1.00**	
Risk persists in ex-users	**3-5yrs**	**1.25**	
	>=6yrs	**1.50**	
C3 As C2, with no risk in ex-users			
Endometrium			
E Protection increases with			
duration of use	**<=1yr**	**1.00**	
Persists in ex-users	**2yrs**	**0.70**	
	>=3yrs	**0.40**	
Ovary			
O1 Protection increases with			
duration of use	**<=2yrs**	**0.70**	
Persists in ex-users	**3-4yrs**	**0.60**	
	5-9yrs	**0.40**	
	>=10yrs	**0.20**	
O2 As O1, with protection in ex-users Remaining for 15 years only			

*The bold rows were included in the standard set of assumptions. * The sources of the relative risk assumptions are discussed in the text.*

Table 3: Assumptions about cancer risk used in the model.

Name	Description	Disease	Relative risk	
			Current-users	Ex-users
CVD1	High risk in current users	AMI	5.0	1.0
	No risk in ex-users	CT	5.0	1.0
		VT	8.0	1.0
		SAH	2.0	1.0
CVD2	**Low risk in current users**	**AMI**	**1.5**	**1.0**
	No risk in ex-users	**CT**	**2.0**	**1.0**
		VT	**4.0**	**1.0**
		SAH	**1.5**	**1.0**
CVD3	Low risk in current users	AMI	1.5	1.25
	Risk persists in ex-users for			
	AMI and SAH	CT	2.0	1.0
		VT	4.0	1.0
		SAH	1.5	1.5

The bold row was included in the standard set of assumptions. *The sources of the relative risk assumptions are discussed in the text.

Table 4: Assumptions about cardiovascular disease risk.

Cardiovascular disease. The main set of risk assumptions for cardiovascular disease (CVD2 in Table 4) was based on results from the *WHO Collaborative Study of Cardiovascular Disease and Steroid Hormone Contraception.* From these, we took a relative risk of 4.0 of death from venous thromboembolism in current users.[4] The WHO study showed an overall relative risk of 3.0 for stroke, but 2.0 seemed more plausible for women in the UK.[12] The relative risk of subarachnoid haemorrhage was taken as 1.5.[13] The WHO study[14] showed a relative risk of 5.0 for acute myocardial infarction. Again, this seemed implausibly high for the risk profile of women currently using COCs in the UK and we therefore used a lower figure of 1.5. However, the higher risk was explored with a second set of assumptions (CVD1 – high risk in current users but no risk in ex-users). We also considered the impact of a low risk in current users with, for acute myocardial infarction and sub-arachnoid haemorrhage alone, a persistent risk to ex-users (CVD3) (Table 4).

Method of analysis. An 'other cause' death rate was calculated by subtracting from the all cause death rate the death rates for the five cancers, for the four cardiovascular diseases, and for maternal mortality, as well as deaths attributed to intra-uterine devices and sterilisation.

The cause specific death rates were then adjusted by the relative risk assumptions according to the pattern of COC use. A standard set of assumptions was used, consisting of L2, B1, C2, E1, O1, and CVD2 (highlighted in Tables 3 and 4). The 'standard pattern of use' was taken to be pattern B: COCs from age 16 to 29, intra-uterine devices from age 30 to 39, sterilisation at 40 (highlighted in Table 2).

In the initial analysis, the standard set of assumptions was combined with the standard pattern of use, assuming the lower contraceptive failure rates. In further analyses, the assumptions were varied for each disease in turn. The standard set of assumptions was also tested against the higher contraceptive failure rates and against the four other patterns of use. A total of 23 combinations of risk assumptions and patterns of use were explored.

Changes from previous model. The model differs from that published previously[2] in four main ways:
- ⑦ We have taken account of new information on breast cancer risk and on the risk of various cardiovascular diseases [4,12-14]
- ⑦ We have made new assumptions about IUD failure rates
- ⑦ We have extended the sensitivity analysis in the model by incorporating new assumptions about the risks of liver, ovarian and cervical cancers and of cardiovascular disease
- ⑦ We have extended the sensitivity analysis in the model by considering the impact of women using COCs continuously from 16 to 49 years.

Results

The numbers of excess deaths in the COC cohort compared to the control group to ages 50 and 75 are shown in Tables 5 and 6 respectively. Based on the standard pattern of use and standard risk assumptions, the number of deaths in the COC cohort at age 50 was 1.7 per cent higher than in the control group. (On varying the risk assumptions this ranged from no change to an increase of 3.8 per cent). This absolute increase of 1.7 per cent in the number of deaths corresponds to an extra 465 deaths by age 50 in a group of one million 16 year old women. Another way of expressing this result is to say that for every 2150 (1000000/465) women starting COSs at 16, one would have died by age 50 because of COC use. (On varying the risk assumptions, this 'number needed to harm' ranged from infinity to 950). To age 75, the number of deaths in the COC cohort was 0.5 per cent lower than in the control group with standard risk and standard use assumptions. That corresponds to a 'number needed to benefit' of 735. (For every COC use.) On varying the risk assumptions, this ranged from a decrease of 1.7 per cent (a number needed to benefit of 207) to an increase of 2.6 per cent (a number needed to harm of 138).

						Assumption				
	Control	Standard	L1	B2	B3	C1	C3	O2	CVD1	CVD3
Liver	125	+392	0							
Breast	4.491	+118		+52	+188					
Cervix	968	+182				0	+31			
Endometrium	49	-30								
Ovary	937	-741						-345		
AMI	749	+10							+82	+192
CT	247	+18							+74	+18
VT	427	+197							+460	+197
SAH	923	+48							+97	+460
Total COC-related	8,914	+496	+105	+430	+566	+16	+47	+891	+931	+1,087
Other	18,762	-8	-5	-7	-9	-4	-4	-9	-15	-12
Maternal	38	-22								
IUD	199	0								
Sterilisation	40	0								
ALL	27,953	+465	+78	+400	+535	-10	+20	+859	+894	+1,053
% change		+1.7	+0.3	+1.4	+1.9	0	+0.1	+3.1	+3.2	+3.8

Table 5: Excess deaths to age 50 in COC cohort compared to control cohort, on various risk assumptions.

						Assumption				
	Control	Standard	L1	B2	B3	C1	C3	O2	CVD1	CVD3
Liver	1,185	+4,109	+4							
Breast	25,715	+138		+73	+207					
Cervix	2,999	+1,501				+4	+35			
Endometrium	1,221	-732								
Ovary	8,651	-6,911						-366		
AMI	32,890	+56							+114	+8,032
CT	13,952	+39							+89	-55
VT	4,666	+203							+464	+178
SAH	3,808	+51							+98	+1,888
Total COC-related	95,086	-1,546	-5449	-1,606	-1606	-2,947	-2,947	4,652	-1,147	+8,004
Other	186,548	+208	+639	+220	+220	+407	+401	-555	+127	-753
ALL	281,910	-1,360	-4,832	-1,408	-1,408	-2,562	-2,540	+4,048	-1,043	+7,228
% change		-0.5	-1.7	-0.5	-0.5	-0.9	-0.9	+1.4	-0.4	+2.6

Table 6: Excess deaths to age 75 in COC cohort compared to control cohort, on various risk assumptions.

	Pattern of use				
	A	B	C	D	E
Liver	0	+392	+392	+392	+391
Breast	+34	+118	+302	+631	+1,067
Cervix	+482	+482	+482	+481	+481
Endometrium	-30	-30	-30	-30	-30
Ovary	-559	-741	-741	-741	-741
AMI	+4	+10	+27	+72	+372
CT	+6	+18	+35	+52	+246
VT	+110	+197	+300	+152	+1,278
SAH	+27	+48	+74	+151	+459
Total					
COC-related	+75	+496	+842	+1,460	+3,523
Other	-4	-8	-12	-17	-27
Maternal	-13	-22	-37	-83	-112
IUD	0	0	0	0	0
Sterilisation	0	0	0	0	0
ALL	-58	+165	+793	+1,360	+3,385
% change	+0.2	+1.7	+2.8	+4.9	+12.1

Table 7: Excess deaths to age 50 in COC cohort compared to control cohort, on various patterns of use.

	Pattern of use				
	A	B	C	D	E
Liver	+3	+4,2092	+4,108	+4,105	+4,091
Breast	+79	+138	+315	+632	+1,820
Cervix	+1,505	+1,501	+1,499	+1,497	+1,488
Endometrium	-731	-732	-732	-732	-734
Ovary	-5,181	-6,911	-6,913	-6,913	-6,918
AMI	+103	+56	+62	+88	+295
CT	+52	+39	+52	+61	+214
VT	+122	+203	+304	+453	1.267
SAH	+33	+51	+76	+151	+451
Total					
COC-related	-4,014	-1,546	-1.228	-659	+1,974
Other	+457	+208	+148	+44	-450
ALL	-3,557	-1,360	-1,118	-698	+1,412
% change	-1.3	-0.5	-0.4	-0.2	+0.5

Table 8: Excess deaths to age 75 in COC cohort compared to control cohort, on various patterns of use.

Pattern of COC use	Breast cancer risk assumption					
	B2		B1		B3	
	50	75	50	75	50	75
A	12	60	34	80	58	104
B	52	73	118	138	188	207
C	146	167	303	320	467	481
D	323	333	632	635	951	947
E	666	995	1,068	1,824	1,470	2,665

Table 9: Number of excess breast cancer deaths to ages 50 and 75 in COC cohort compared to control cohort, on various patterns of use.

Different patterns of use. Tables 7 and 8 show how the number of deaths varied with different patterns of COC in use, assuming the standard set of risks. The total number of deaths varied with different patterns of COC use, assuming the standard set of risks. The total number of deaths in the COC cohort compared to the control group ranged from an increase of 0.2 per cent to an increase of 12.1 per cent to age 50, and from a decrease of 1.3 per cent to an increase of 0.5 per cent to age 75.

Risk of breast cancer. Table 9 shows the effect on the number of breast cancer deaths to ages 50 and 75 of different patterns of COC use and of different risk assumptions. Although the possible variation in breast cancer risk is clearly important, within the ranges of assumptions examined in the model, the number of deaths was clearly more sensitive to the effect of varying patterns of use.

Contraceptive failure rates. Analysis of the standard set of assumptions against the standard pattern of use resulted in 22 fewer maternal deaths in the COC cohort than in the control group. Doubling the contraceptive failure rates resulted in 45 fewer maternal deaths in the COC cohort than in the control group.

Discussion

Within the model, over the range of assumptions about the relative risk of diseases associated with COC use and about the patterns of COC in use, the number of excess deaths at ages 50 and 75 in the COC cohort was not large compared to the control group. This provides some reassurance about the likely adverse effects of COCs.

The results of this analysis cannot be readily compared with those of the earlier model,[2] despite the similarity of approach. There are two main reasons for this. First, we have used more up to date, cause specific death rates (which may show both temporal changes for particular diseases and also, in the case of the cancers, artefactual changes due to changes in rules governing the coding of death certificates[9]). Second, we have updated the assumptions used about the relative risk of death associated with COC use. In particular the degree of uncertainty about the risk COC use is associated with a definite but modest increase in risk.[8]

Limitations of this approach. The model describes the risk profiles of individual women in a way that is unavoidably crude. For instance, it does not take into account the complexity of women's reproductive lives, and in particular the varied and discontinuous use that women make of contraceptive techniques. Nor does it consider the possible effect of other risk or protective factors for the diseases considered: smoking, high blood pressure, cervical screening and so on.

As a guide to expected changes in mortality, the model also has a number of important limitations. First, the cancer mortality rates applied to the control group were derived from the experience of a population with many women alread y using COCs. In our earlier model,[2] we used mortality rates from 1970-1972, years when we hypothesised that COCs would have had little effect on cancer mortality. However, to use such dated vital statistics no longer seems appropriate. Second, the relative risks of breast cancer mortality that we used were calculated from a meta-analysis that looked at the incidence of, rather than mortality from, the disease. Since the excess cancers diagnosed tend to be less advanced clinically, the number of excess breast cancer deaths estimated in the model is likely to be an overestimate. Third, nearly all the impact on mortality that we estimated derives from the relative risks observed with COC preparations which are older than those currently used.

Despite these limitations, the model clarifies the relative importance of different causes of death in ways that illuminate the public health impact of COCs and might be helpful to individual women when they are making contraceptive choices.

Varying relative risk assumptions. Breast cancer is the most important cause of death to age 50 in both the COC and control groups, accounting for roughly half of the deaths from COC related causes (Table 5). However, the number of excess deaths in the COC cohort was small, even with the worst case assumption (B3). Cervical cancer was the second, but much less common, cause of death, with COCs producing a 50 per cent increase in the number of deaths from this cause. If, however, the risk does not remain elevated in ex-users (C3), then there were very few excess deaths. The protective effect of COC on endometrial cancer was small because of the low incidence of the disease. However, the effect of COC use on ovarian cancer deaths until 50 was important, even where protection is assumed to last for 15 years only (O2).

Subarachnoid haemorrhage and acute myocardial infarction were important causes of death to age 50, but even on the high risk assumption the effect of COC use is not great. However, when an elevated risk in ex-users was assumed (CVD3) the number of excess deaths is greatly increased. The effect of varying assumptions about venous thromboembolism is also clear. A low risk assumption brought about a 50 per cent increase in deaths, but the high assumption doubled the number of deaths compared to the control.

The differences between the impact of COCs at ages 50 and 75 were crucially dependent on the effects of earlier COC use on death rates from ovarian cancer, myocardial infarction and subarachnoid haemorrhage. The model shows that the COC group experienced fewer deaths overall to age 75 on all assumptions except O2 (where the protection against ovarian cancer remained only for 15 years), and for CVD3 (where the risk in current users was low but remained in ex-users).

An area not considered here in depth is the possible contrast in health effects between second and third generation progestogens. The WHO study showed that venous thromboembolism was more than twice as common in women using one of the third generation drugs gestodene or desogestrel) as in women using levonorgestrelo.[5] This finding (similar results have been reported elsewhere [6,7]) has received a lot of publicity and was taken into account with the 'high risk' set of assumptions in the model (CVD1). However, these findings are based on relatively small numbers of women and so are necessarily imprecise. Moreover, there are beneficial metabolic changes associated with the third generation drugs and the intriguing possibility has been raised by the WHO study (based on only eight patients) of no increased risk at all in SMI risk for women using these drugs.[14] Given so much uncertainty, it would not have been appropriate to have explored this contrast further with the model.

Varying patterns of COC use. Although the patterns of COC use examined are clearly artificial, they highlight an important point. That is, that varying patterns of COC use may have a greater impact on the final result than varying assumptions about the relative risk of particular diseases.

Pattern A, for instance, produced the fewest deaths at both ages 50 and 75. The increase in the number of deaths from cervical cancer and cardiovascular disease compared with the control cohort were roughly balanced by the reduction in the number of deaths from ovarian cancer. Pattern E, on the other hand, produced the largest number of excess deaths, brought about by increased breast cancer and CVD deaths. These contributed to its being the only pattern with more deaths to age 75 than the control cohort.

Conclusion

These results highlight the need for further research, in two areas. First, more needs to be known about the effects of COCs in ex-users, particularly in women over 60: how long do the beneficial and harmful effects associated with their use last? Second, we need a clearer view of past, present and possible future patterns of COC use: what are the implications of these for lifetime risk of the diseases associated with COC use?

More immediately, the results of the model call into question current advice to women that it is safe to continue using COCs until the menopause, in the absence of certain other risk factors. If longer duration of use, particularly into a woman's 40s, is indeed associated with a larger number of excess deaths, there may be implications for contraceptive advice. The response to the recent venous thrombosis scare shows that women are sensitive to new evidence about risk and are prepared to make changes to their contraceptive use.

References

1. Vessey, M.P. The Jephcott Lecture. 1989. In: Mann, R.D. ed. *Oral contraceptives and breast cancer.* Parthenon Publishing Group. 1990, 121-132.

2. Milne, R., Vessey, M.P. Modelling the impact on mortality of the use of combined oral contraceptives. *Br.J. Family Planning,* 1991: 17: 34-38.

3. Dillner, L., Controversy rages over new contraceptive data. *Br. Med. J.* 1995: 311: 1117-1118.

4. World Health Organisation Collaborative Study of Cardiovascular Disease and Steroid Hormone Contraception. Venous thromboembolic disease and combined oral contraceptives: results of international multi-centre case-control study. *Lancet.* 1995: 346: 1575-1582.

5. World Health Organisation Collaborative Study of Cardiovascular Disease and Steroid Hormone Contraception. Effect of different progestagens in low oestrogen oral contraceptives on venous thromboembolic disease. *Lancet.* 1995: 346: 1582-1588.

6. Jick, H., Jick S.S., Gurewich, V. *et al*. Risk of idiopathic cardiovascular death and nonfatal venous thromboembolism in women using oral contraceptives with differing progestagen components. *Lancet.* 1995: 346: 1589-1593.

7. Spitzer, W.O., Lewis, M.A., Heinemann, L.A.J. *et al*. On behalf of Transnational Research Group on Oral Contraceptives and the Health of Young Women. Third generation oral contraceptives and risk of venous thromboembolic disorders: an international case-control study. *Br. Med. JK.* 1996. 312: 83-88.

8. Collaborative group on hormonal factors in breast cancer. Breast cancer and hormonal contraceptives: collaborative reanalysis of individual data on 53 297 women with breast cancer and 100 239 women without breast cancer from 54 epidemiological studies. *Lancet.* 1996: 347: 1713-1727.

9. Office of National Statistics. *Mortality statistics. Series DH2 no. 21.* London: HMSO, 1996.

10. Office of National Statistics. *Birth statistics. Series FM1 no. 23.* London: HMSO, 1996.

11. Ory, H., Darroch Forest, J., Lincoln, R. *Making choices evaluating the health risks and benefits of birth control methods.* New York: The Alan Guttmacher Institute, 1993.

12. World Health Organisation Collaborative Study of Cardiovascular Disease and Steroid Hormone Contraception. Ischaemic stroke and combined oral contraceptives: results of an international multi-centre, case-control study. *Lancet.* 1996. 348: 498-505.

13. World Health Organisation Collaborative Study of Cardiovascular Disease and Steroid Hormone Contraception. Haemorrhagic stroke, overall stroke risk and combined oral contraceptives: results of an international, multi-centre, case-control study. Lancet. 1996: 348: 505-510.

14. World Health Organisation Collaborative Study of Cardiovascular Disease and Steroid Hormone Contraception. Acute myocardial infarction and combined oral contraceptives: results of an international multi-centre case-control study. *Lancet.* 1997: 349: 1302-1209.

Resource 2

John Sneddon

Chemistry revision

The structure of atoms

All matter is composed of atoms and each atom is made up from three smaller particles. These are the protons and neutrons that form the central nucleus of the atom, and electrons. Protons carry a positive electrical charge, represented by +, and electrons carry a negative charge, represented by - ; neutrons do not have a charge.

The electrons in an atom move rapidly around the nucleus and are arranged in shells – each shell containing a fixed number of electrons. When atoms combine together to form matter the atoms in matter are held together by forces of attraction known as chemical bonds.

There are two types of chemical bond: the covalent bond in which the atoms share the electrons in their outer shells and the ionic bond in which an atom either loses or gains an electron. In this revision we will only look at the ionic bond.

A good example of a molecule that is made up of two atoms held together by ionic bonds is salt (sodium chloride). Sodium (Na) atoms have a total of 11 electrons: two in the first shell, eight in the second and one in the third. Chlorine Cl atoms have 17 electrons: two in the first shell, eight in the second, and seven in the third shell. Because eight electrons are required to fill both the second and third shells this means that sodium has one electron too many to fill the second shell and chlorine has one electron too few to fill the third shell. If we put sodium and chlorine together to form sodium chloride then sodium can give up its spare electron to chlorine to complete its third shell. This reaction can be shown in the following equation:

 + Cl   + Cl

As a result of sodium 'giving away' an electron to chlorine the outer shell of each atom is filled with the correct number of electrons, but now each atom is unbalanced as far as their electrical charges are concerned.

ACTIVITY   ALLOW 5 MINUTES

If sodium gives up its single electron what will that do to the electrical charge on the sodium atom? Write your answer below.

Commentary

Sodium now has 10 electrons but it still has 11 protons present in the nucleus. This will give it a net electrical charge of +1 which is represented as Na^+.

ACTIVITY   ALLOW 5 MINUTES

If the chlorine atom receives the electron from sodium, what will this do to the electrical charge on the chlorine atom? Write your answer below.

Commentary

When the chlorine atoms accepts the electron it will now have 18 electrons. However it will still have 17 protons in the nucleus and therefore has a net charge of –1. This is represented as Cl^-.

Each of the charged atoms represented by Na^+ and Cl^- are called ions.

Molecules can behave like atoms and those that do donate or accept can form ions. This property is important when we come to explain the movement of drugs across cell membranes.

Positively charged ions such as Na^+ are called cations.

Negatively charged ions such as Cl^- are called anions.

A salt is made up of a cation and an anion, with the exception of the hydrogen ion H^+ or the hydroxyl ion OH^-.

In the solid state, ionic bonds in a molecule are relatively strong and the compound stays as a solid. However, when dissolved in water, the ionic bonds in many compounds are weakened. In many compounds they are so weak that the ions that make up the compound separate and create a solution which consists of a mixture of free positively-charged and free negatively-charged ions. When this happens we say the compound has ionised or that the compound has become dissociated.

The fact that many chemical compounds become dissociated in water is essential to a living organism because then the ions are free to take part in chemical reactions within the body. From the point of view of pharmacology and drug action, almost all drugs are active only after they have dissociated into ions at their site of action.

REFERENCES

GOODMAN and GILMAN (1990) *The Pharmacological Basis of Therapeutics*, Pergamon Press.

LEHNE, R.A. (1995) *Pharmacology for Nursing Care*, 2nd edition, W. B. Saunders & Company.

SPENCER, R.T., NICHOLS, L. W., LIPKIN, G.B., HENDERSON, H.S. and WEST, F.M. (1993) *Clinical Pharmacology and Nursing Management*, 4th edition, J B Lippincott & Company, Philadelphia.

TROUNCE, J. (1993) *Clinical Pharmacology for Nurses*, 14th edition, Churchill Livingstone.

WALKER, R. and EDWARDS, C. (1994) *Clinical Pharmacy and Therapeutics*, Churchill Livingstone.

WHITE, A. (1994) 'Pharmacology for nursing practice', *British Journal of Nursing*, 3, 506–509.

GLOSSARY

Agonist –
a drug that binds to receptors and activates them into producing a measurable response

Antagonist –
a drug that binds to receptors but does not activate a response

Biotransformation –
alteration of chemical compounds by the enzyme systems of the body

Clearance –
the rate of removal of a drug from the body

Clinical pharmacology –
the study of the action of drugs in humans

Compartment –
organs, tissues, cells and fluids in which the uptake and distribution of a drug is identical

Drug –
a chemical that affects living tissue

Endocrine chemical signalling –
hormone secreting cells secrete their chemical messengers directly into the bloodstream

Enzyme induction –
an increase in enzymic activity resulting from exposure to any of a wide range of chemical agents

Excipient –
inactive constituent of a pharmaceutical preparation

Extent of absorption –
the amount of a drug absorbed by the body following administration

First-pass effect –
partial metabolism of a drug by the liver before it reaches the site of action

Gap junction –
'holes' in the cell membranes between two cells through which the cytoplasms of the cells can make contact

General sales list medicines –
drugs which may be sold from outlets other than pharmacies

Medicine –
a mixture of one or more drugs, combined or formulated with excipients

Metabolites –
the breakdown products of a drug

Neurotransmitter –
chemical messenger within the autonomic nervous system

Paracrine chemical signalling –
chemical transmission between paracrine cells which release a local hormone and tissue cells close to the paracrine cell

Pharmacodynamics –
the effect that drugs have on the human body

Pharmacokinetics –
the process of drug absorption, distribution and final elimination from the body

Pharmacology –
knowledge of the history, source, physical and chemical properties, compounding, biochemical and physiological effects, mechanisms of action, absorption, distribution, biotransformation and excretion, and therapeutic and other uses of drugs

Pharmacy medicines –
drugs sold to the public without a prescription by a pharmacist from registered premises

Prescription only medicines (POMs) –
drugs sold or supplied only in accordance with a prescription given by an appropriate practitioner

Pro-drug –
conversion of a drug to its active compund by enzymic activity

Rate of absorption –
the time taken for a drug to leave its site of administration

Receptor –
a specialised receiving agent located on the cell surface

Signalling molecule –
molecule which influence the behaviour of other cells with which it has direct contact

Synapse –
a specialised gap or junction at nerve endings across which chemical transmission takes place

Synaptic chemical signalling –
chemical transmission between the cells in the nervous system and between nerve cells and other cells such as muscle cells

Therapeutics –
the medical use of drugs

Volume of distribution –
a measure of the distribution of water in which a drug has become distributed within the body